The Addicted SOUL

The World of Addiction

Internet, Gambling, Drinking,
Shopping, Texting …

Stories, Information and
Spiritual Guidance

Rabbi Dovid Goldwasser

ISBN 978-1-60091-197-2

Book design by Avrohom Kay

Published by:
Israel Bookshop Publications
501 Prospect Street
Lakewood, NJ 08701

Tel: (732) 901-3009
Fax: (732) 901-4012
www.israelbookshoppublications.com
info@israelbookshoppublications.com

Printed in the United States of America

Distributed in Israel by:
Shanky's
Petach Tikva 16
Jerusalem
972-2-538-6936

Distributed in Europe by:
Lehmanns
Unit E Viking Industrial Park
Rolling Mill Road,
Jarrow , Tyne & Wear NE32 3DP
44-191-430-0333

Distributed in Australia by:
Gold's Book and Gift Company
3- 13 William Street
Balaclava 3183
613-9527-8775

Distributed in South Africa by:
Kollel Bookshop
Ivy Common
107 William Road, Norwood
Johannesburg 2192
27-11-728-1822

Table of Contents

< 3 >

< 4 >

< 5 >

בס"ד

ברכת מרן הגר"ח קנייבסקי שליט"א

———————

בעזה"י

בערב ש"ק לסדר אז ישיר משה, דברנו עם
הגאון הדור מורינו הרב חיים שליט"א,
אודות הספר 'נפשי בשאלתי' והיה מאד
מרוצה והשיב בשמחה ברכה והצלחה.

וכשביקשו ממנו מהו הדעת תורה אודות
התמכרות ענה:

מיט שכל קען מען ארויסקריכען פון דעם.

[תרגום חפשי ללשה"ק: בהשכל ובדעת יש לצאת
מזה.]

הסכמת הרה״ג רבי ישראל הלוי בעלסקי שליט״א
ראש ישיבה ישיבת תורה ודעת

ישראל הלוי בעלסקי

לכבוד הרה״ג ר׳ דוד גאלדוואסער שליט״א

עברתי בעיון רב על החיבור היקר ״נפשי בשאלתי״
לתועלת אלה הנדבקים והקשורים לאיזה רעל נפשי
המשעבד אותם ומקלקל את נפשם - ומה שקורין
היום Addiction, וכמעט שאבדה להם הבחירה
והדעת העצמאית לעשות כרצונם הטוב. והנה
הקוראים האומללים ימצאו בעי״ה דרך סלולה בספר
הנוכחי והדרכה מועלת מאד, ועצות נכונות היאך
להמילט מהפח שנלכדו בו רח״ל, ולאוהביהם ימצא
שביל איך להציל את ידידיהם ולהעמידם על דרך
סלולה וישרה ואנה ואנה ילכו עם בעיותיהם ואנה ימצאו
העצה וההדרכה הנכונה.

אפריון נמטייה להרב ר׳ דוד על דבריו הנעימים ועל
עוד חבוריו המועילים ויזכה לחיי אושר והצלחה על
אשר הביא תועלת גדולה למבקשי הדרכה.

יום ח׳ לחודש שבט תשע״ב לפ״ק
ישראל הלוי בעלסקי

RABBI MOISHE STERNBUCH

CHIEF RABBI

and Vice President of
the Orthodox Rabbinical Courts
Jerusalem

•

Rechov Mishkalov 13 Ilar-Nof Jeruslaem Tel:02-651-9610

משה שטרנבוך

ראב"ד

לכל הקהלות האשכנזים

מח"ס מועדים וזמנים ושו"ת תשובות והנהגות
רב בית הכנסת הגר"א, ור"מ במרכז התורה הר-נוף
סגן נשיא העדה החרדית
בעיה"ק ירושלים ת"ו

בעזה"י

לכבוד הרב דוד גאלדוואסער שליט"א, רב דקהלת בני יצחק, ומרביץ תורה
לאלפים.

על דבר שאלתכם בענין האינטרנט למיניהם ובפרט בהמשך לשיחתנו
ע"י הטלפון, הנני משיב מפני הכבוד, התורה הקדושה אמרה כמעשה
ארץ מצרים אשר ישבתם לא תעשו וכמעשה ארץ כנען אשר אני מביא
אתכם שמה לא תעשו ובחקותיהם לא תלכו, ופי' רש"י "מגיד שמעשיהם
של מצריים ושל כנעניים מקולקלים מכל האומות", כלומר אף שכל האומות
מקולקלים הם במעשיהם אמנם של מצריים ושל כנעניים מקולקלים יותר
מכל שאר האומות.

ביאורן של דברים, ארץ מצרים באותה תקופה היתה ידם בכל, היו יושבים
ברום העולם כולם היו נכנעים מפניהם, כל כסף וזהב אשר בארצות באו
להם, היו יושבים על סיר הבשר, ועל דרך זה אנשי כנען בעת שבאו ישראל
לרשת את הארץ היו הכנעניים המושלים בתבל וכמו שאמרו חז"ל שלכל
מלך ומדינה הי' להם נציג בארץ כנען, לעומת זה ישראל עם קרובו היו
מתי מעט ואפ"כ נצחו שלא כמנהג העולם, ולמה, מדינות הללו היו שטופים
בעריות ובזנות, ובמקום טומאה אין קיום, מזהיר התורה הקדושה כמעשה
ארץ מצרים אשר ישבתם בה וכמעשה ארץ מצרים אשר מביא אתכם שמה
אם אתם רוצים לזכות לבוא לארץ ישראל צריכים להתנהג בקדושה, סוד
קיום של עם ישראל הוא התנהגותן בקדושה.

כהיום אשר אומות העולם השיגו כל מיני התקדמות בטכנלוגיה באופן בלתי
משוער מנתיחה על הלבנה עד הפלא הפלא פלפון פחות משיעור ג' על ג', עם כל
זה בחרו להשתמש עם זה להרבות טומאה ורציחה בעולם, דברים אשר
לא שערום אבותינו [ולכן אנו רואים מפעם לפעם טרגידיות שנוגעים לאלפי
ורבבות ולדוגמא ניקח ההר-געש אשר קרה במדינת אירופא ובכל העולם
סבלו מהתוצאות].

בעזה"ר האינטרנט רבים חללים הפילה, העצה היחידה ללחום נגדה
ולהסתתר מפניה הוא להתחזק עם התורה ומצותיה, ורק בזה נזכה לשמירה
מעולה מאת הבורא ברוך הוא.

בכבוד הרב משה שטרנבוך

ראב"ד דבד"צ עדה החרדית

מכתב
מאת הגאון הצדיק פאר דורינו,
מרן רבי אביגדור מיללער זצללה"ה

ב"ה

כבר נתפרסם הרב דוד גאלדוואסער במעשיו
הרבים כאיש הרוח מדריך בני אדם בדרך
התורה, ועכשיו מוסיף גם בחיבורו זה ללכת
בדרכו לעורר ולעודד ולפתח נשמת חיים
בקרב רבים מבני עמנו. יצליחהו ה' בכל מעשיו
ויפוצו דברי השפעתו בישראל.

נאום

אביגדור הכהן מיללער

מכתב ברכה ועידוד זה קיבל הרה"ג המחבר שליט"א ממרן הגה"צ
רבי אביגדור הכהן מיללער זצללה"ה זמן קצר טרם הסתלקותו לחיי
עוה"ב, והוא א' ממכתביו האחרונים שכתב בעצמו, ברוב חביבותו
למורנו המחבר שליט"א, לכן אמרנו להדפיס המכתב כאן.

Acknowledgments

Hagaon Rav Aharon Kotler notes how great is the obligation of a person to constantly reflect upon and recognize the good that Hashem has done for him. This will bring the individual to an elevated level in *bitachon*, because he will perceive the Divine Providence that guides his life.

I humbly thank Hashem for giving me the privilege to be involved in many different endeavors on behalf of the *klal*. It is through some of this work that I have had the opportunity to meet precious *nefashos*, some of whose stories are included in this book. May Hashem grant me the wisdom and insight to continue helping His children and to bring glory to His Name.

To Martin E. Friedlander, Esq., whose keen interest and expert help in every aspect of this book is responsible for its publication. He is a unique leader whose vision for the future has guided countless individuals and organizations and has expanded Torah horizons beyond imagination. It is my privilege to have his partnership in so many worthwhile undertakings. May Hashem grant him continued *hatzlacha* and *bracha* in all his endeavors.

My heartfelt appreciation to my colleagues and friends in the medical and mental health community, whose understanding of and sensitivities to the observant population is heartening. Their cooperation and collaboration in facilitating treatment have been gratifying.

< 14 >

The pen is too feeble an instrument to adequately thank Mrs. Simi Eichorn for all her work. The Al-mighty has blessed her with unusual *kochos,* and I thank her for sharing them with the *klal.* The numerous projects that I have been involved in over the years all bear her imprimatur.

To Rabbi Moshe Kaufman of Israel Bookshop Publications for all of his efforts on behalf of the *klal.* His vision, initiatives and insights have truly enhanced the field of Jewish publishing. May he have continued *bracha v'hatzlacha* in all of his efforts *l'hagdil Torah ul'ha'adirah.*

To R' Moshe and Rivky Moskowitz for their extraordinary support and dedication to the *klal.* May they have great *nachas* from their outstanding children, Effie, Yitty, and Ezra.

To R' Avrohom Kay, whose brilliant artistic ability has enhanced Jewish publications throughout the world. Over the past two decades it has been a *zechus* for me to work together with him on so many different endeavors.

To Rabbi and Mrs. Yosef Stamm for their dedication to this project. Their *yedidus* and participation in every book is a great source of *chizuk* to me. May they continue to be *marbeh kevod shamayim* through their many activities on behalf of the *klal* till 120.

To Dr. and Mrs. Shimon Frankel for their devotion to the *klal* and for their involvement in this publication.

With deep appreciation to R' Duvy and Miriam Kramer, *mokirei rabbanan,* for helping to raise the bar of *chashivus haTorah.* Their *hishtatfus* in this volume is a great source of personal encouragement. May they continue to have much *nachas* from their outstanding *mishpachah.*

With special thanks to Mr. Jerry Greenwald, Mrs. Naomi

< 15 >

Mauer, and Mr. Steve Walz of the Jewish Press.

To Nachum Segal, renowned radio personality, a master of words and an eloquent spokesman for Klal Yisrael. It has been a privilege to work together with R' Nachum for over twenty-five years. His unique talents and efforts have united people from all walks of life.

Special thanks to R' Eliezer and Gitty Allman, Eddie and Helene Appelbaum, Rabbi Yosef Gesser, Rabbi Shmuel Grossman, Rabbi Moshe Kolodny, Sonja Samokovlija, and Howie and Rochelle Sirota.

Forever etched in my *neshamah* is the selfless dedication of my beloved parents, R' Yitzchak ben R' Yeruchem and Riva Tzirna bas R' Benzion z"l, as well as the *mesiras nefesh* of my esteemed father-in-law, R' Chaim Baruch ben HaRav Elimelech z"l. May the example of their noble lives always serve as a source of inspiration and blessing.

To the honored matriarch of our family, Mrs. Esther Koval, who carries on the royal lineage of the distinguished Kovalenko and Fink families.

To my *eishes chayil*, Hinda Chaya, whose wisdom, insight, fortitude and understanding are a wellspring of *chizuk* for our entire *mishpacha*. בית והון נחלת אבות ומה' אשה משכלת. May we merit much *nachas* from our children and our grandchildren as they follow in the footsteps of their great ancestors.

המצפה לישועת ה'
Rabbi Dovid Goldwasser

< 16 >

Introduction

W E LEARN IN *PARSHAS KI SISA* THAT AFTER SPENDING 40 DAYS and nights in Heaven, Moshe Rabbeinu descended to witness the scene of *chet ha'egel* (Sin of the Golden Calf) and he broke the *luchos* (the Tablets). Subsequently, he ascended for another 40 days and nights, following which he came down with a second set of *luchos*.

HaGaon HaRav Moshe Feinstein asks: Why did Moshe Rabbeinu need to spend an additional 40 days and nights together with Hashem? He had already learned the contents of the Torah and the manner of instruction during the first 40 days he spent in *Shamayim* (Heaven).

Rav Moshe answers that one cannot compare the spirit and moral fiber of Bnei Yisrael before the *chet ha'egel* to the world that existed after the *chet ha'egel*. It was no longer the same world. It would be more difficult for Moshe to lead a generation that had made breaches. It would be necessary to increase their will, to promote their fortitude, strengthen their courage, and inspire their character. Now another, alternative approach and an entirely different methodology would be required in order to teach the Torah to Bnei Yisrael.

The world of the 21st century is, indeed, a new world. We are living in different times that demand a new understanding and awareness of the mindset and attitudes of the generation. The issues and challenges of today are overwhelming and threaten the core of our survival as a Jewish nation. It is crucial that we grasp the severity and dangers that exist, so that we can comprehend the course of action that is most helpful and effective in combating the problem.

< 17 >

Some of the addictive behaviors are, in truth, recurrent and familiar. What is worrisome, though, is the development of new insidious dependencies that jeopardize not only one's physical wellbeing, but the spiritual welfare and safety of many. Often the individual does not even discern how deeply entrenched he has become in his "habit."

The great R' Chaim of Sanz, known as the Divrei Chaim, thoughtfully gazed out at the street and saw a Jewish person walking by. He quickly tapped on the window and asked the gentleman to come in.

"What would you do," he asked the man, "if you found a chest full of silver and you knew to whom it belonged? Would you return it?"

The Jew answered, "Of course, I would return it immediately."

R' Chaim was disappointed with his answer and said, "You're a fool!"

Soon another Jew passed by his window, and R' Chaim invited him in and posed the same question to him.

The second man responded, "Do you think I'm a fool to return such a precious treasure?"

R' Chaim told him, "You are wicked."

R' Chaim waited until he espied a third passerby. Once again R'Chaim tapped on the window and invited the gentleman in. "What would you do," he asked the man, "if you found a chest full of silver and you knew to whom it belonged? Would you return it?"

The third Jew thought for a moment and then said, "Rebbi,

< 18 >

I don't know what I would do if I found such a treasure. It is possible that Hashem would help me withstand the challenge. Perhaps I would be able to fight my *yetzer* (Evil Inclination), resist the temptation to keep it, and return the treasure to its rightful owner. But there is also the possibility that I will fail and keep the treasure for myself. Since I have not been challenged with this *nisayon* (challenge) it is difficult to know what I would do."

"You are a wise man," said R' Chaim, "and you have given a clever answer."

Our generation is engulfed by a myriad of *nisyonos* which do not discriminate among their victims. Some people are under the false impression that they are impervious to specific challenges, such as those covered in this book, and they have nothing to be concerned about.

Unfortunately, my experience within the community over the past decade clearly indicates that there is no immunity against these *nisyonos* that are out there. The *yetzer* does not offer anyone preferential treatment, exemption, or a free pass, and often people have been drawn into a life of long-term addiction from a single misstep. Many of my counseling sessions with individuals have been increasingly focused on the various addictions addressed in this book.

One can never predict how he/she will react or cope with the challenge when it presents itself. As we travel through the corridor of life, challenged by pitfalls, traps and obstacles, it is important to be educated and aware of the dangers that lurk. Addiction is insidious and creeps up on people, slowly overtaking their lives. As the saying goes, "Forewarned is forearmed," and there is no more apt truism with regard to addictions.

I have had many requests from *mechanchim*, community

< 19 >

leaders, parents and siblings to offer a resource on this topic
and to provide guidance in a public forum.

This book is written to communicate a deeper understanding of the world of addictions and its challenges, as
well as to delineate coping methods and an effective road to
recovery. It is a valuable "escape route," whether one is already caught in the grip of an addiction or, alternatively, one
is searching for ways to protect himself from falling prey to
an addiction. For those already caught in the grip of an addiction, the first step toward recovery is the recognition and
admission that one is unable to disassociate from his "habit."
It is not an easy matter to extricate oneself from the clutches
of such dependency. For all others, it is important to analyze
the progression of these ills and to develop the appropriate *gedarim* (safeguards) to protect oneself from, perhaps, the
greatest *nisyonos* of our generation.

ויהי רצון מלפניך ה' אלקינו ואלקי אבותינו

שתרגילנו בתורתך ודבקנו במצותיך,

ואל תביאנו לא לידי חטא

ולא לידי עברה ועון

ולא לידי נסיון ולא לידי בזיון ...

And may it be Your will, Hashem, our G-d,
and the G-d of our forefathers,
that You accustom us to study Your Torah
and attach us to Your commandments.
And do not bring us into the hands of error,
nor into the hands of transgression and sin,
nor into the hands of challenge,
nor into the hands of scorn ...

< 20 >

Internet/ Computer Addiction

< 21 >

Internet/Computer Addiction

In Tehillim (140:8) David HaMelech asks Hashem to "protect my head on the day of armed battle... " One of the explanations offered by the Talmud Yerushalmi (Yevamos 78a) is that this verse refers to the battle of Gog and Magog.

HaGaon HaRav Elazar Shach cites the Ponovezher Rav who asks: Why did David HaMelech request protection specifically for his head, more than any other part of his body? After all, when one is afraid of the dangers of the battlefield, every limb and organ is vulnerable to attack.

His explanation sheds light upon the battles we are waging on a daily basis – in our communities, in our homes, and in our hearts. David HaMelech foresaw that preceding the arrival of Mashiach there would be an intense conflict with Gog and Magog. Moreover, their weapons of war would be unusually destructive and would be targeted to damage the "head."

David HaMelech was, in fact, not referring to physical danger, but rather to a spiritual threat. This is the threat we are contending with in these times of technological progress.

< 23 >

Danny's Story

It was a blustery Motzoei Shabbos, right after *Havdalah,* when I first heard Danny's panicked voice over the telephone.

"Rabbi Goldwasser? Is this Rabbi Goldwasser?"

"Speaking."

"I don't know if this is a good time or if I'm imposing... I must talk with you about a very urgent matter .... Could I make an appointment, like, right now?"

I invited him without hesitation, and the young man promised to arrive momentarily. The doorbell clanged less than ten minutes later.

"*A gutte voch,*" I greeted him. "Come in and warm up a little."

The young man, did not identify himself and gratefully stepped inside, slowly removing his snow-covered coat.

"I'm Danny G.—" he began quietly. "I...Uh, there's something I wanted to discuss. Actually, a better word would be 'confess'. Yes, there's something I have to confess."

My heart went out to this earnest young man who appeared not a day older than twenty-one. Something was pressing on him, clouding his expressive eyes with shame and regret.

"I'm one of five children in a *frum* family," Danny said, after we sat down in my study. "Like my brothers, I traveled the regular route of a yeshiva education. I was just one of the boys, growing and learning and letting off steam."

His voice trailed off into silence; his discomfort was

< 24 >

palpable. Aware of his distress, I waited patiently for him to collect his thoughts and proceed with his narrative.

He continued, "It was only recently that I veered off in a different direction. I finally acknowledged that learning didn't come easily to me and I would probably be better off in a different environment. Several months ago, I began working at an entry-level position in an established corporation."

The picture that emerged was that of a *frum* young man, who had chosen a path that he felt was more suitable for himself. His obvious anguish remained a mystery.

"Rabbi Goldwasser, I'm not a strong learner. When I come home from work, I've got nothing to do. Many of my *chaverim* are already married, so I'm often at loose ends. I'm feeling a little unfulfilled at times."

The distress he currently displayed seemed to have been set off by some cataclysmic incident.

By now Danny was nervously twisting a piece of paper he had picked up into an array of geometric shapes, breathing deeply in an effort to steady his voice. When he resumed speaking, an air of resignation had settled over him.

"A short while ago, a co-worker introduced me to a new, enthralling occupation. A toy, he called it. He showed me how to surf the Internet and I was hooked immediately. I devoted my free time to this captivating pursuit," Danny softly explained. "There were so many opportunities for social networking; for expanding my horizons. I joined on-line dialogues and became a regular participant in the numerous discussion groups that thrive on the Internet."

A sense of foreboding came over me, as I realized that Danny's insecurities made him a prime target for the unseen

< 25 >

predators of the twenty-first century. Danny fell silent, and I knew, without a doubt, that the worst was yet to come.

"It was this past Erev Shabbos when I realized that the Internet is not a toy. It's a weapon and I, an inexperienced warrior, foolishly took this weapon into my own hands! I came home from work at about 2:00 p.m., and I knew that there was still plenty of time before Shabbos. In my quiet, private apartment there wasn't much to do in terms of clean-up and preparation. With more than two hours to go before sundown, I logged onto the Web."

Questions hovered at the tip of my tongue, but I restrained them. This was Danny's story, and he would tell it at his own pace.

"Rebbi, when I glanced up from the screen I realized that... I saw the hands on the clock. They had moved three hours ahead while I was glued to the screen. Three hours!"

His narrow shoulders trembled at the memory, but he forced himself to continue speaking.

"Shabbos had come in and I had been oblivious," he cried. "I was never *mechalel* Shabbos [desecrated the Shabbos] before in my life. *Never!* And now, because of a mindless pursuit, I had done the unthinkable. Sitting in front of the screen, I felt like a total failure."

Guilt and regret flickered in Danny's eyes. In my mind's eye, I pictured him sitting glancing at the clock above his desk. Could one fathom the pain – the humiliation – of violating the Shabbos due to mere oversight?

"What did you do after that?" I asked gently.

"I rushed over to my parents' home," Danny continued. "I

< 26 >

told them that I had fallen asleep in *shul*, and they accepted my excuse. But you know, and I know, that this glib response was far from the truth."

His head bowed in shame, his body heaved as he cried and groaned, "Not only did I not *daven* [pray] that Friday night and lie to my parents. I was *mechalel* Shabbos! I feel trapped and am fearful for my spiritual future...."

● ● ●

< 27 >

As a Rav in the community, and as a consultant to communities around the world, I have seen the devastating effects the Internet has had on individuals, families and even communities. Much has been said about its dangers and potential pitfalls, yet its tentacles continue to extend into the very hearts of our insulated communities.

It's an ironic twist of language that terms one an Internet "user," in the same vein as a drug addict who is universally dubbed a "user." Is it any wonder that this global social hall has been termed the "web," evoking the image of one who has been caught in its tenacious grip and finds it very difficult to extricate himself without outside assistance?

At this time, surfing the Internet has far exceeded the problematic halachic and hashkafic issues that are involved, as it has commandeered the time and attention of many individuals to the exclusion of everyone and everything else.

The disorder of Internet addiction is a compulsive impulsive disorder that should be considered a psychological ill. It is estimated that 9 million people in America could be labeled "pathological computer users."

HaGaon HaRav Michel Yehuda Lefkowitz (1913-2011) remarked, *"Kol hachurban bizmaneinu hu al yedei ha'internet* – the destruction and decadence that we are witnessing in our times is due to the Internet." When I met with him about a year before his *petirah* I informed him that his words had made a deep impression on many individuals, and he was very pleased that his message had been disseminated and had made an impact.

We recite twice daily in the *Krias Shema*, *"V'lo sasuru acharei levavchem v'acharei eineichem* – you shall not explore after your heart and eyes." The plethora of sites that provide unlimited information in the category of the three cardinal sins – *avodah zarah, shefichas damim* and *giluy arayos* (idolatry, murder and

< 28 >

immorality) makes it extremely difficult for many to contain their curiosity and refrain from inspecting these sites. Yet our sages have taught us that whatever the eye sees, even for a short time, makes an indelible impression on one's psyche. There is no easy way to expunge that imprint.

The *pasuk* tells us *(Bereishis 9:23)*, "And Shem and Yafes took a garment, put it on both their shoulders, and they walked backwards and they covered their father's [Noach's] nakedness; their faces were turned away, and they did not see their father's state of undress."

Rabbi Yechiel Yehoshua Rabinowicz, the Chelkas Yehoshua (1766-1813), comments on the apparent repetition in the *pasuk*. It is stated initially "*vayelchu achoranis* – they walked backwards," which implies that their faces too were backwards, yet the *pasuk* continues, "*upneihem achoranis* – and their faces were turned away."

The Chelkas Yehoshua notes that it was not sufficient for Shem and Yafes to merely turn away their faces or close their eyes in this situation. They had to actually turn their back and their faces so that they should not in any way experience the sight of their father's state of undress.

The Chelkas Yehoshua observes that if we would be as vigilant to guard our eyes from that which we should not see then many of the *tzarros* of our times would not occur.

The Medrash tells us that the sin of the *dor hamabul* (the Generation of the Flood) originated with a deficiency in guarding their eyes, as we learn *(Bereishis 6:2)*, "*Vayiru bnei ha'elohim ...* – the sons of the princes and judges saw that the daughters of man were good and they took themselves wives from whomever they chose." Rashi explains that they conducted themselves in ways that would make a person's hair stand on end.

< 29 >

The commentaries tell us that the eyes are a gift from HaKadosh Baruch Hu. How could a person use Hashem's gift to sin? It is compared to a king who bequeaths his servant with a gift, which the servant then proceeds to disgrace.

Our eyes are a generous present from Hashem which we must care for and protect.

The Sochachover Rebbe (1838-1910), known as the Avnei Nezer, notes that the eyes are the gates to the heart. He explains that man's heart is generally influenced by what he sees with his eyes. Thus, one who exerts every effort to only look at good things will inherently be a good person. One who is indiscriminate, however, bares his soul to random stimuli that exist in the world.

The Divrei Shmuel comments on the Talmud's prohibition of looking at the image of an evil person *(Megillah 28a)* that gazing at such a picture creates a connection and a bond between the two.

The son of R' Chaim Zeitchik, who was one of the leading *gedolim* in Yerushalayim, related the following incident that took place on Chol Hamoed Pesach.

"My father, who had a weak heart, became very ill during Chol HaMoed Pesach and desperately needed his medication. The local pharmacies were already closed. I made a number of calls until one of my acquaintances told me that a pharmacy located on Rechov Yaffo remained open at night. He happily offered to go and came over immediately for the prescription.

"My father, however, would not allow him to go. He said he didn't want to trouble the young man, but he insisted it was no trouble at all. Then I suspected that perhaps my father thought that the situation was not so serious and didn't want to take the medication, so I explained to him that it was a matter

< 30 >

of *pikuach nefesh*. My father remained adamant and would not let the man go.

"I continued to beg my father to let him go get the medication from the pharmacy. Finally my father relented and said to me, 'I will tell you the truth. I know where this pharmacy is located and it is almost impossible for one to guard the *kedushah* (holiness) of one's eyes. I would not want to cause any individual to do any wrong on my account.'"

Only after R' Zeitchik was reassured and promised that the young man's spiritual welfare would not be compromised and there would not be any risk did he agree to let the young man go to the pharmacy and get him the medication he needed.

The anonymity and ease of accessibility to the Internet from the privacy of one's own home has eliminated any element of shame or indignity. It offers irresistible entrée to a world many people might not have been brave enough to enter.

The Hegyonah Shel Torah comments on the anomaly presented in *Parshas Noach*. He notes that Cham, the son of Noach, was deemed worthy to be saved from the Flood. Yet, upon emerging from the *teivah*, when Cham found his own father intoxicated and lying without clothes, he made fun of him and ridiculed him. It is difficult to understand how a son could so dishonor his own father in his moment of weakness, yet have been judged deserving to be spared the fate of his generation.

It is explained that, indeed, Cham would never have committed such a despicable act before the Flood, because society would have condemned him for the offensive behavior. Now, due to the annihilation of the Flood, only Noach's immediate family existed, and Cham was no longer concerned about public disapproval or humiliation.

< 31 >

Similarly, those wishing to engage in illicit or inappropriate behaviors no longer have to venture out into the public arena and chance censure or reprimands.

Not only is there anonymity when one surfs the Internet, but one also enjoys a sense of disengagement which is liberating. People don't interact with each other in real time, for example on Facebook and MySpace, and don't have to deal with anyone's response to something they said or "posted." This is known as the "disinhibition effect" which allows individuals to say and do things in cyberspace they wouldn't ordinarily say or do in real life.

< 32 >

Zoe's Story

Zoe, a 20-something young woman from the midwest, had moved to New York and worked in a corporate office in the city. In order to meet new people, she posted her profile on Facebook and joined the social networking community in cyberspace.

Zoe's network grew and she eventually made the acquaintance of a young man. Their relationship progressed and they soon became officially engaged. Of course, their engagement was posted online; their Facebook status was no longer "single."

It was disconcerting to Zoe, though, when she found inappropriate messages posted on her fiance's Facebook wall. However, since the social networking sites are public domains it is virtually a free-for-all, and Zoe's fiancé denied any association or friendship with whoever was sending him messages.

Plans were set in motion for a wedding in a few months, and Zoe blithely drafted lists of wedding halls, caterers, gown designers, and the myriad of arrangements that would have to be made.

One morning when she walked into her office, the usual chatter suddenly halted in mid-sentence and the office was deathly quiet. Taken aback, Zoe cried out, "What happened?"

Her co-workers gazed back at her sadly, but silently, until she could no longer bear it. "Please tell me what is wrong!" she pleaded.

Zoe's colleague who sat in the adjoining cubicle in the large office space came running over to her and said, "We are so sorry."

< 33 >

Zoe looked at her blankly. "Why are you consoling me?"

She then learned that her fiancé had broken up with her on Facebook. Instead of talking to her in private, Zoe's fiancé had chosen to announce his decision in this public forum. He just "put it out there" and avoided the need to offer any explanations or invest any personal emotions.

Zoe, on the other hand, was mortified. Her family, her friends, her co-workers, the people she cared about most and even those she hardly knew, had all witnessed her public disgrace and shame.

• • •

< 34 >

Louis J. Freeh (Director FBI, 1993-2001) testified before Congress about the dangers to children and stalking on the Internet. Children and teens often become victims of cyber-bullying – where they are harassed, humiliated or otherwise targeted by their peers who post mean notes on websites or post personal information meant to embarrass another child. When an adult is involved it is termed cyberstalking or cyber-harassment and has more significant legal ramifications. In addition, there are literally tens of thousands of pedophiles in cyberspace, who prey on children using the Internet, and there is little security and/or protection.

Of course, many feel that the storehouse of information that is made accessible by the Internet overrides any concerns that are voiced. Shlomo HaMelech states in *Koheles (1:18)*, "*Yosef da'as, yosef ma'achov* – the more knowledge, the more pain." The acquisition of information has not come without a price, and the price that some have paid has been devastating.

The Talmud recounts *(Nedarim 9b):*

אמר (רבי) שמעון הצדיק מימי לא אכלתי אשם נזיר טמא אלא אחד
פעם אחת בא אדם אחד נזיר מן הדרום וראיתיו שהוא יפה עינים וטוב
רואי וקווצותיו סדורות לו תלתלים אמרתי לו בני מה ראית להשחית
את שערך זה הנאה אמר לי רועה הייתי לאבא בעירי הלכתי למלאות
מים מן המעיין ונסתכלתי בבבואה שלי ופחז עלי יצרי ובקש לטורדני
מן העולם אמרתי לו רשע למה אתה מתגאה בעולם שאינו שלך במי
שהוא עתיד להיות רמה ותולעה העבודה שאגלחך לשמים מיד עמדתי
ונשקתיו על ראשו אמרתי לו בני כמוך ירבו נוזרי נזירות בישראל

> *Shimon HaTzaddik once stated, "In all*
> *my days I never ate of the Asham offering*
> *of a Nazir* who became tamei (ritually*
> *unclean), except for one. There was a*
> *Nazir from the south who had become*
> *ritually unclean. I saw that he had*
> *beautiful eyes and was good-looking. His*

< 35 >

*hair was beautifully arranged in curls. I
said to him, 'My son, why did you find it
necessary to destroy this beautiful hair of
yours?'*

*(*A Nazir is one who voluntarily abstains
from drinking wine and cutting his hair,
and avoids contact with the impurity
associated with death, for a period of at
least 30 days.)*

*"He replied to me, 'I was a shepherd in
the city where I lived. I once went to fill a
pail of water from the well, and I saw my
reflection in the water. At that moment my
Evil Inclination overtook me and wanted
to banish me from the world [by bringing
me to sin]. I said to the yetzer hara: You
wicked one, why are you arrogant in a
world that is not yours with a person who
in the future will be consumed by the dust
of the earth? I swear by the Temple that I
shall shave you for the sake of Heaven.'*

*"Immediately I stood up and kissed him
on his head. I said to him, 'May there be
many more like you who undertake a vow
of Nezirus in Israel like you.'"*

The Bais Yisroel comments that Shimon HaTzaddik
inquired of the *nazir:* What did you see that you found it
necessary to destroy your hair? Why would a person like you
have to worry about the *yetzer hara* (Evil Inclination) to the
extent that you had to accept upon yourself *nezirus?*

The *nazir* replied: Even absolute *tzaddikim* can be defeated.
It happened to me that the *yetzer hara* assailed me. I was only

< 36 >

saved when I took immediate action and swore that I would cut off my hair for the sake of Heaven."

It is clear from here that the *yetzer hara* is so powerful that even the most righteous person can fall prey. One cannot delude himself into believing that he/she is immune to any malevolence, or addiction, associated with Internet usage.

< 37 >

Shmiel's Story

A Yid, Shmiel, called me early one Sunday morning that he had a private matter he needed to discuss with me as soon as possible. Although I was available in the afternoon, he insisted that he could only come late at night, and he finally agreed to come at 10:00 that evening.

When I opened the door at 9:45, I was surprised to see an elderly man who appeared to be in his mid-70s standing nervously in the doorway. I welcomed him in, and after a few moments of uncomfortable silence, I gently prompted him to tell me the reason for his visit.

His discomfort increased and he became agitated. I was reluctant to press Shmiel and waited until finally he began, albeit hesitantly.

"I have a computer in my home." Silence.

"And?" I questioned softly.

"I learned how to use it, and I am able to visit many sites." Again there was silence.

Hemming and hawing, Shmiel continued, "I met somebody …. In one of the chat rooms… We have been corresponding …. I finally spoke to her on the phone." There was a long pause, and then he said, "I have an appointment to meet her."

"What would you like from me?" I asked, dreading the answer.

Shamefacedly, he explained that he is married, with children and grandchildren. Nobody knows about his treacherous activities on the Internet. He is overcome with pangs of guilt, and knows that he would be thoroughly humiliated and dis-

< 38 >

graced if anyone ever found out. "But," he protested, "every moment on the Internet is so thrilling. I have never enjoyed myself so much.

"What shall I do?" he cried.

Shocked by his revelation, I told him that, quite frankly, he should consider himself fortunate that, with *siyata d'shmaya*, he had regained his good judgment and stepped back for a moment.

I instructed him to immediately sever any contact with the woman. I then advised him to contact someone for professional counseling the next morning and to undertake a program of learning to fortify his spiritual wellbeing.

The elderly Yid was flabbergasted. "How will I continue to live?" he cried. He had been feeling useless and inadequate and this contact had revitalized him and filled a gap in his life, he remonstrated.

I slowly tried to draw him back to reality by quoting Chazal (*Sotah 3a*), "Reish Lakish said: A person does not commit a transgression unless a spirit of craziness *(ruach shetus)* enters into him." I pointed out that the *yetzer hara* is so compelling that it has the ability to undermine one's rational power of reasoning. I begged him to reconsider his foolish behavior and reminded him that he would lose the respect and love of his wife and family. He would be a pariah in the community.

I repeated my recommendations that he enlist a strong support/counseling system to guarantee his full disassociation from the computer and any outside relationships.

The elderly Yid finally consented to follow through on my advice and we set up a system so that he could report to me on his progress.

< 39 >

After the Yid left, I sat and pondered this disconcerting incident. It was shocking that a "respectable" person of such an advanced age had been caught in the web of the Internet.

The Tiferes Uziel comments on the *pasuk* in *Yeshayah (1:18)*, "If your sins are like scarlet, they will become white as snow ..." and notes that if a young person sins it is tolerable, since his passions are strong. But, "There are four people the mind cannot tolerate: A poor man who is arrogant, a wealthy man who flatters, a lecherous old man, and a community leader who shows off without cause" *(Pesachim 113b)*. Consequently, if a person transgresses in an age appropriate manner there is hope for him – his sins can become white as snow. But if an individual is debauched, and conducts himself in a manner that is totally inappropriate for someone his age, what hope is there for him?

• • •

< 40 >

According to a British study (Shotton, 1989), many cannot resist exploring the Internet as they find it an appealing alternative to real life. Contrary to humans, the computer is logical, predictable, and – perhaps most importantly – not judgmental. Computer addicts have a narcissistic relationship with their computers and form emotional bonds to them.

The Satmar Rebbe, HaRav Yoel Teitelbaum, once chastised an individual who wanted to stay in a hotel overlooking the beachfront. The man protested that only those who wish to look will do so. "On the contrary," replied the Rebbe, "if one **can** look then he **wants** to look."

People using the Internet are exposed to ultra-violent games, satanic worship, racist propaganda, hate talk, recipes for manufacturing drugs, instructions on how to commit suicide and directions on how to make bombs.

It is common knowledge that there is a profusion of websites set up by cult and missionary groups, with many specifically targeted at a Jewish audience. Some of these sites are so cleverly disguised that the unsuspecting surfer often does not even realize that the site is not sponsored by a legitimate Jewish organization/individual. Hebrew words are used, complete with Jewish symbols and quotes from so-called rabbis. Passages in the Torah as well as Jewish customs are presented and discussed – for the express purpose of confusing people and entrapping them.

The Torah tells us (*Devarim, 13:18*), *"V'lo yidbak b'yadcha me'uma min hacherem* – no part of the banned property may adhere to your hand." The Talmud *(Makkos 22a)* derives from this prohibition that it is forbidden to have any benefit from *avodah zarah*. This prohibition extends to all the related aspects of *avodah zarah* which one is proscribed from bringing into his domain.

< 41 >

A number of years ago I was invited to address a meeting of prominent *askanim* (community leaders), with members of the general public in attendance, concerning the rising threat of missionary and cult groups who target the Jewish community. When I left the gathering, a teenager was waiting outside and asked if he could speak to me for a few minutes. He said that he had heard my presentation, but could not see anything wrong with being involved with missionary groups.

It soon became very clear that the young man was highly intelligent and had already developed very strong feelings about a particular missionary group. I was curious how the relationship had evolved, and the teenager explained that he had been bothered by many questions about man's purpose in this world and his relationship with G-d. He immediately tapped into the most available resource about spirituality, right in his own home: the Internet. He found a site that seemed to fit the bill perfectly.

He posted his initial inquiry, and received a quick response, which was then followed up by aggressive outreach workers who used a number of methods, including "love-bombing," to try and hijack his *neshamah*.

It was way back then, yet, on that cold night in December, when I was forced to face the sad realization that the cyber-world was light years ahead of some of our human efforts to inculcate our youth with Torah values and hashkafos. The danger has only increased manifold and its destruction is non-discriminatory.

It should be noted that many do not even realize how far things have already gone in this area. We have a direct command in the Torah (*Devarim* 7:3), "*Lo tischatein bam* – nor shall you enter into marriage with them." The Ramban (*Tur Shulchan Aruch, Even Ha'ezer 16*) explains all the halachic ramifications of this particular command.

< 42 >

Risa's Story

Unfortunately, I became privy to such a tragedy a few years ago when I received a call from the Shomrim (an organization of volunteer Jewish civilian patrols that work together with law enforcement personnel) who serve our community in many ways. They wanted me to speak to the distraught parents of a girl who had been reported missing.

I climbed up four flights of stairs to a small apartment that was cooled only by a revolving stand fan, and met with the parents who had emigrated from Hungary a few years ago. Risa's mother couldn't speak; she sat at the small kitchen table and moaned softly. Her father was heartbroken, and he explained that he and his wife worked extremely long hours to provide for their three children. Risa's father toiled in a bakery approximately twelve hours each day, rising before 5:00 AM every morning. But, he sighed, he never complained about the hours of back-breaking work because he felt he was doing it all for the benefit of his children. He and his wife wanted to offer their children all the opportunities they never had in their country of origin.

He had taken great pride in his oldest daughter, Risa, who had become a star student in school. He and his wife had been looking forward to seeing much nachas from her as she made great strides in all her studies. The father noted that Risa didn't bring home many friends, but he had attributed that to her embarrassment of the family's apparent poverty. Nevertheless, he asserted, in order to assure the children's firm adherence to Yiddishkeit, he had not placed them in public school. Despite the expense, all his children were in Beis Yaakov schools.

In the past few months, he had been especially pleased to see how studious Risa had become. She spent hours on her computer working on school assignments. He was gratified

< 43 >

to know that his years of hard work were finally beginning to pay off.

Then, just a day earlier, Risa disappeared without a trace. They called a few of her friends they did know, they spoke to the school administration and her teachers, but nobody had a clue. Finally, this morning, they had received a tip from an anonymous caller who suggested that they check her computer files.

An expert was brought in who was able to hack into her computer system. The girl had been visiting many chat rooms, joining the hundreds of thousands of individuals who participate in this social networking. Combing through her e-mail correspondence revealed that a serious relationship had developed online between the teenage girl and a non-Jewish man living in Chicago, leading to the "missing girl" situation. The correspondence between the two confirmed that Risa had run away from home to join her "cyber friend" in Chicago.

The appropriate authorities and the FBI were contacted in order to locate Risa. It took a while until she was tracked down. Thankfully the relationship had worn a little thin, but it still took some time before she could be extricated and the family was reunited.

• • •

< 44 >

Facebook is all the rage, and no less popular within our own community. Its appeal as a social networking website is global. The ability to connect with friends and their friends' friends is intriguing for every teenager, young adult, business person, etc.

Facebook users create a profile page that contains contact information and personal details about themselves which everyone within their network can view. From the time the individual signs up at this social site he begins to add friends to his network. The set of connections grows as each friend adds his own group of friends to this same network. Eventually many of the "friends" who have joined the network are really not well known to anyone.

It is common for relationships between boys and girls to develop among Facebook users. While such a phenomenon is less threatening to the general population, such a trend is anathema to the Jewish community and leads, in due course, to the transgression of many *issurim* (Torah prohibitions). Unfortunately, many in our community are still naïve and think that computer relationships can't go very far. Regrettably, there is nothing further from the truth.

HaGaon HaRav Shlomo Wolbe was asked the following question 20 years ago (before any awareness of the computer's pervasive negative effects on one's spirituality).

A benefactor had offered to donate computers for all the students of a boys' yeshivah for after-school activities.

The Mashgiach advised them to refuse the contribution for two reasons:

He explained that the boys' mission in life is to become *talmidei chachamim*. They have to apply themselves to learning. The computer was addictive; the boys could become totally

< 45 >

absorbed in the computer and lose any chance of future greatness in Torah. It is well known, he observed, that it is impossible to support two addictions simultaneously.

Secondly, he noted, the interpersonal character traits of a child are established at a young age. It is important for children to engage in play and communication with others. That is when children learn how to be forgiving, how to compromise, how to share and be tolerant. A child who spends his free time immersed in his computer and masters it, tends to prefer that activity rather than playing with others. He soon loses any interest in engaging in proper social interaction.

It should be noted that in those days Rav Wolbe still did not know the extent and severity of the problems that would result from the worldwide web, but he already foresaw with his sagely wisdom its inherent dangers.

Sue Palmer, author of *Toxic Childhood* and *Detoxing Childhood* (pub. 2006 and 2007, respectively), and a former headteacher in Scotland, discusses the negative aspects of screen-based entertainment and notes: "We are seeing children's brain development damaged because they don't engage in the activity they have engaged in for millennia … I'm not against technology and computers. But before they start social networking, they need to learn to make real relationships with people."

The *Washington Post* has called the Internet the largest repository of obscene material in the history of mankind. These sites on the Internet have their own devastating effect on the moral fabric of society.

Studies indicate that use of the Internet is a significant factor in nearly 50% of all familial and/or marital relationship problems. In the past, children and couples would spend evenings and free time together, talking and/or playing

< 46 >

games. Internet addiction or compulsive use of the computer has changed those dynamics. The Internet addict becomes entrenched in his unhealthy behavior to the point of social isolation, disrupting his academic or job performance, and/ or causing the spouse and families to seek counseling for relationship problems.

Experts note that Internet addiction replaces food, sleep and earning a living for many addicts. Children don't sleep at night in pursuit of their computer compulsion. Parents stop relating to each other and spend less time raising their children. Over the years, there have been stories in the news of mothers who neglected their children in pursuit of their obsession with the computer.

It is interesting to note that after Chava had partaken of the fruit of the *eitz hada'as,* she justified her lapse by saying *(Bereishis 3:13),* "The serpent deceived me and I ate."

Hashem had specifically commanded Adam and Chava, "of the Tree of Knowledge of Good and Bad you must not eat thereof ..." Our sages explain that the serpent, i.e. the *Satan,* was persuasive. The argument was that at most she would only be transgressing one *aveirah.* Chava could never have imagined that merely eating from the fruit of the *eitz hada'as* would change her entire life as well as the future course of Klal Yisrael.

Similarly, the computer is perceived as a wonderful innovation, granting access to the information highway, i.e. the Internet, a treasure trove of knowledge and learning that can enrich one's life. Yet, it is indeed a "tree of knowledge of good and bad." Does anyone conceive of the possibility that the introduction of the computer into his home may radically change lives, and not for the better? The thought may cross one's mind that a transgression may perhaps be committed, deliberately or unwittingly, but most never consider the reality that it may destroy their life, their home, and the lives of others.

< 47 >

In addition, violence is equally available on the Internet with a similar negative effect on society. Our *gedolim* have commented on the damaging influence of being exposed to violence. (See *Be'er Moshe*, Section 4, 147: 21- 22; *Yabia Omer*, Section 1, *Orach Chaim* 7.) A Harvard psychologist, Ronald G. Slaby, was quoted in the *National Review* (1993) that "the impact of viewing violent images causes young people to experience a victim effect, (increased fearfulness) and a bystander effect (increased callousness and desensitization to violence)."

It should be noted that clinicians and researchers who testified before the Senate Commerce Committee's Science, Technology and Space Subcommittee in November 2004 described the immorality on the Internet as "the new crack cocaine," with similar destructive results.

One should never delude himself into believing that he is beyond temptation and that he can control his *yetzer hara.* Chazal tell us *(Kesubos 13b)*, "No one is immune from the possibility of having improper relationships."

Researchers and advocates of Internet safety are constantly beseeching Congress to enact stronger laws to ensure that children, especially, are not exposed to the obscene material which floods the Internet and has grown to epidemic proportions. Studies show that 7 out of 10 children access these sites inadvertently, and one in three have done so intentionally. Statistics show that the average age of exposure is 11 years old – some start at 8 years old. Current data indicates that a total of 4.2 million websites, or 12% of the total number of websites, contain obscene material. It is reported that every second 372 Internet users are typing in adult search terms into search engines and 28,258 Internet users are viewing these sites.

It is important to note at this point that, with the advent of blogs on the Internet, an entirely new genre of *lashon hara,* that

< 48 >

is troubling and alarming, has been introduced into our lexicon.
A blog is a website where everyone can write everything they
please about anyone and anything. It is a public forum that
gives any and every individual a voice that is heard throughout
the world.

Many blogs are, in essence, online diaries created by
teenagers in which a considerable amount of personal details
is included. This leaves them open to the potential dangers of
cyberstalking by adult strangers and cyberbullying by peers.

Other bloggers include frustrated, and even disturbed,
individuals who have time on their hands and choose to freely
spew their vitriol about an individual, an organization, a
corporation, or something/somebody in the news. Many have
a personal axe to grind and are on a witch hunt – identified in
the 21st century as cause-stalking or blog bullying.

"In an abundance of words sin will not be lacking, but one
who restrains his lips is wise," says Shlomo HaMelech *(Mishlei
10:19)*. Certainly when individuals – each with his own agenda
– decide to express their cynical and derogatory opinions even
about *gedolei Yisrael* (Torah leaders), there is great cause for
concern and righteous anger.

Generally, there is an overwhelming admiration in today's
community for *talmidei chachamim* and *gedolei Yisrael*. However,
the accessibility of the Internet and the uninhibited exchange
of bloggers articulating their personal thoughts and feelings
allow a minority of individuals to malign the reputation of
our Torah leaders. Protected by the anonymity of their screen
names, in the privacy of their homes and behind closed doors,
there are individuals who have a need to engage in self-
aggrandizement by belittling our *talmidei chachamim* (Torah
sages) and promulgating blatant *lashon hara* and *hotza'as shem ra*.
"Cursed is the one who strikes his brother in secret," adjures the
Torah *(Devarim 27:24)*. Rashi says that this refers to one who has

< 49 >

spoken *lashon hara*. The actions and remarks that are discussed on these blogs are most often slanderous and a complete falsification of facts. The entire discussion is actually scorning the word of Hashem Himself.

The Talmud *(Sanhedrin 99b)* tells us how great is the punishment of one who infringes on the honor of our Torah sages. Yet, notes the Chofetz Chaim in *Hilchos Lashon Hara,* the *yetzer hara* uses his wiles to convince a person that this admonition is not relevant in today's times and only applied in the era of the great *Tanna'im* and *Amora'im.*

There is nothing further from the truth, states the Chofetz Chaim, for each *talmid chacham* is assessed according to the generation in which he lives. Thus, in our days a person who engages in Torah learning all day, or one who teaches others Torah, is considered a *talmid chacham.* An individual who humiliates or debases a *talmid chacham,* even in a general way, has committed an egregious transgression. The Talmud *(Shabbos 119b)* states that there is no remedy for one who dishonors a *talmid chacham.*

Furthermore, the one who listens to *lashon hara* – or in the case of bloggers, reads the *lashon hara* – is equally liable for the transgression of *lashon hara.* Our sages tell us that it is forbidden to accept or believe *lashon hara* and by listening, i.e. reading it, one might cause himself to believe it. This is forbidden regardless of the subject and regardless of the writer.

We learn that one of the reasons the *Beis HaMikdash* was destroyed was because the people of that generation humiliated the *talmidei chachamim (Shabbos 119b).*

Internet sites of reputable organizations and Jewish media that allow unsupervised discussions on their blogs bring down the standards of *kavod chachamim* and *emunas chachamim.* There needs to be a public outcry for accountability and

< 50 >

effective monitoring of blogs; alternatively, the blogs should be withdrawn or discontinued.

A distinguished *posek* once rendered a halachic decision, which was publicly attacked on a popular blogsite by one of his detractors. The blogger alleged that the *psak* had been wrongly issued and was a miscarriage of justice.

The *posek* was asked, "Doesn't it bother you that your *psak* is being challenged in such an underhanded way?"

The Rav answered, "Not at all. I am only distressed that there is an individual who is so unconcerned about being a *chote u'machati es harabim* and goads others to transgress the sin of *lashon hara*, all in the name of Torah."

Bringing the Internet into the home poses serious questions of *"lifnei iver lo sitein michshol* – you shall not place an obstacle in front of a blind person." Causing another Jew to sin is an *aveirah*. (See *Igros Moshe, Orach Chaim 3:43; Shevet Halevi, 4a.*) Even if one is willing to take responsibility for his own *aveiros*, one certainly does not wish to be a *chote u'machati es harabim* – one who sins and causes others to sin.

The lure and fascination of the Internet is thus very challenging to many individuals on a variety of levels.

< 51 >

Yehuda's Story

A while ago I received a call from an influential *askan,* a pillar of his community in Long Island. He stated that he and his 11-year-old son had a pressing issue to discuss with me. I picked up a note of angst in his voice, and I agreed to see them the next morning.

After exchanging friendly greetings and a handshake, the father of the young boy quickly cut to the chase.

"Yehuda and I have a *sheilah* (halachic question) and we would like to consult *daas Torah* as to what we should do.

"Yesterday afternoon," he began, "Yehuda was in the den playing on the computer. Bored of the games he had already played, he had typed in a new search for children's games.

"He was requested to confirm that he was an adult in order to enter the site, so he came out to the yard, where I was sitting and learning, and innocently requested that I sign in for him so he could play on this site."

The man paused, and I was surprised to see that he was sweating profusely. He resumed his tale, but he seemed shaken and overwrought.

"I told him, 'no problem,' but was curious why an adult's confirmation was needed.

"He must have made a small typographical error, because when I went over to the desk and saw the inappropriate site that had appeared on the screen, I almost fainted! Had my child not been so ingenuous, I shudder to think what he would have seen with just one more click!

"I immediately turned off the computer. After I had caught

< 52 >

my breath, I spoke to Yehuda.

"My next step was to call you. I need the advice and *psak* of a Rav. My question is threefold: What is the appropriate response to yesterday's near-disaster? Should the family continue to use the computer for non-business related activities? Should the computer be removed from the house?"

The "tree of knowledge of good and bad" has been brought back in our times. Today, too, the devastating effect of partaking from that which is prohibited continues. A young child is just as predisposed to become Internet addicted as an adult, perhaps even more so.

In this particular instance, *baruch Hashem*, the child, due to his naivete, moved on and was not victimized.

• • •

< 53 >

We say every day in our morning prayers, " Do not bring us into ... the power of transgression and sin, nor into the power of challenge." The Michtav M'Eliyahu notes that people must be challenged in life in order to generate their spiritual growth. What we are asking for is that the *nisyonos*, the challenges, should not be intense or unbearable.

Why do we continue the prayer, *"v'lo lidei bizayon* — and do not bring us into the power of scorn"? Although we may be challenged it doesn't necessarily have to be a source of embarrassment.

It is explained, though, that when an individual fails to successfully meet his challenge he is personally embarrassed and his self-esteem plummets. In addition, it is very possible that – in the case of an addict — his personal failure will become public knowledge and then he will be looked down upon and disdained.

< 54 >

Are You Addicted?

Internet/computer addiction covers a broad gamut of behaviors including an obsession with social networking, compulsive use of online auction sites, compulsive web surfing or database searching, frequenting adult chat rooms, and obsessive playing of offline computer games. The symptoms of Internet addiction vary from person to person, but there are some red flags that would indicate that there is a problem.

- Do you feel more comfortable with your online friends than your real ones?

- How often do you form new relationships with other on-line users?

- Does your time on the computer cause you to neglect your relationships, your work, school or other important aspects of your life?

- Do others complain to you about the amount of time you spend online?

- Do you always check your e-mails before doing anything else?

- Do you think obsessively about being on the computer or playing computer games even when you're involved in other activities?

- Do you lose track of time online?

- Are you annoyed when your online time is interrupted?

- Do you get depressed, moody or nervous when you are off-line, and find that your mood improves once you are back online?

< 55 >

- Do you lie or deceive others about your Internet use, i.e. the extent or nature of your online behavior?

- Do you feel a sense of excitement when engaged in the use of the Internet?

- Do you find you can't stop yourself even when it is resulting in negative consequences in your life?

- Are you losing sleep because of all the time spent online?

< 56 >

Help

Behavior Modification

Keep a log of your Internet activity and then review the information. Try to determine if there are specific times of the day that you are using the Internet more and/or if there are triggers that make you stay online longer than intended.

Implement small incremental steps to modify your Internet use.

Try changing your routine, scheduling a different time of day to go online.

Set a timer to limit your amount of time on the computer.

Turn off your computer at a specified time each evening.

Replace a specific amount of time spent on the Internet with another enjoyable activity that you have turned your back on.

Support System

Enlist friends and relatives to help you moderate your Internet usage.

Develop more meaningful relationships in real life.

Analysis

Explore causal issues that may be feeding your Internet addiction.

Develop strong coping skills that will help alleviate the need to resort to the addictive Internet usage.

< 57 >

Spiritual Help

Prayer

Our sages tell us *(Kiddushin 30b)*, "Were not Hashem to help man he would not be able to prevail."

Tefillah (prayer) was established in order for a person to develop a closer relationship with the Ribono Shel Olam. It is one of the effective modes we have to combat our challenges in life.

Our sages comment on the *pasuk* in *Bereishis (2:5)*, "All the trees of the field were not yet on the earth, and all the herb of the field had not yet sprouted, for Hashem had not sent rain upon the earth ..." They note that although the grass and trees were ready to come out from the ground on the third day, Hashem waited for man to pray for rain before He sent it down and made the plants grow.

It is important for a person to employ the means of *tefillah* to obtain what he needs. What is more, our sages tell us that *tefillah* has the unique power to even enable one to obtain that which he would otherwise perhaps not merit.

Although one may despair and think that since he has descended to such a low spiritual level his *tefillos* will be futile, David HaMelech states *(Tehillim 118:5)*, "*Min hameitzar karasi Kah anani vamerchav Kah* – from the depths I called upon Hashem; Hashem answered me with expansiveness."

Developing an Agenda for Spiritual Growth

The *Shulchan Aruch (Yoreh Dei'ah 203:6)* states that if one is afraid that he will be ambushed by his *yetzer hara* and he will transgress one of the *mitzvos lo sa'aseh*, it is a *mitzvah* for him to swear an oath that he will not succumb to his Evil Inclination.

The *Sefer HaChinuch (Mitzvah 188)* maintains that if an

< 58 >

individual feels that the *gedarim* (boundaries) instituted by Chazal are not sufficient for him, and he will possibly succumb to the *yetzer hara,* he should establish a set of limitations for himself that he feels will be more effective. The *Sefer Yisrael Kedoshim* notes that if a person does transgress he should undertake to pay a penalty. I would recommend that if one visits websites that are not business-related he should, for instance, set aside a specific amount of money for *tzedakah* or he should expend a specified amount of extra time learning Torah.

Establishing Mentor/Chavrusa Program(s)

Shlomo HaMelech tells us in *Koheles (4:9),* "Two are better than one." It is essential for the addict to find a sponsor/mentor. Sponsors are often another addict in recovery who is willing to share the experiences of his journey with the sponsee. He is a source of strength and hope who will enable the addict to recover from his behavioral problems.

It is also advisable for the addict to establish Internet accountability by making arrangements with a support system or installing filtering software that either monitors web browsing activity and reports it to a parent, mentor or Rav or denies access to inappropriate sites, images and messages. There are server-based filters, which are updated at the server, intended to block access to inappropriate material or controls that are offered by the Internet Service Provider (ISP). Some filter providers also offer a closed system option which is probably even safer. The closed system locks one out of the Internet, allowing access only to pre-selected safe Internet sites.

Some of the popular filtering and monitoring programs are listed below:

- **Accountable2you** (reports searches initiated and sites visited) accountable2you.com
- **Eblaster** (reports all computer activities and will also

< 59 >

block sites as requested)
eBlaster.com

- **Jnet** (filter for computer and mobile devices)
thejnet.com

- **K9** (free Internet filter and parental control software)
K9webprotection.com

- **Koshernet** (Internet filter)
koshernet.com

- **NetNanny** (built-in filtering system)
NetNanny.com

- **WebChaver** (logs and reports all web browser activity)
webchaver.org

- **WebSense** (a filtering and reporting system)
websense.com

- **Yeshivanet** (only allows access to selected sites)
yeshivanet.com

According to many *poskim,* if one will incur additional charges in order to put these safeguards in place, he may use his *ma'aser* money to cover the fee.

The importance of this safeguard is highlighted by the Vilna Gaon's commentary on a statement in the Talmud *(Berachos 28b)*. The Talmud relates, "When Rabbi Yochanan ben Zakkai fell ill his disciples went to visit him … They said to him, 'Master, bless us.' He said to them, 'May it be the will of Hashem that the fear of Heaven shall be upon you like the fear of man.' His disciples said to him, 'Is that all?' R' Yochanan ben Zakkai said, 'If only you can attain this! For when a man is committing a transgression he says: I hope no man will see me.'"

The Gaon notes that when talking about man's transgression the Talmud expresses it in the present tense, i.e. the *aveirah* is already being executed. He explains that *yiras shamayim*

< 60 >

is only a deterrent prior to the commitment of an *aveirah*. Once the person is already acting on the *aveirah*, he will only be curbed if someone opens the door and catches him in the act, because then he will be embarrassed and immediately withdraw.

The Vilna Gaon concludes: How great was the blessing of R' Yochanan ben Zakkai that a person's fear of Heaven should be like his fear of man.

In fact, HaGaon HaRav Shmuel HaLevi Wosner *shlita* is quoted *(Sefer Yisrael Kedoshim)* to have said that if Chazal would have had to contend with the Internet in their days they would have instituted an *issur* of *yichud* with the computer, similar to the established prohibition of seclusion of a man and woman. Rav Wosner therefore directed that if one needs to access the computer it would be advisable to do so only when another person is present in the room.

< 61 >

Breaking the Addiction

"Rav Huna said in the name of Rav: Once a man has committed a transgression twice – *avar aveirah v'shanah bah* – it becomes permitted to him. Permitted? How could that come into one's mind? Rather, it appears to him like something permitted." *(Yuma 87a)*

The Satmar Rebbe asks why the Talmud didn't say that the person committed a transgression and then "returned" to the *aveirah* – *avar aveirah v'chazar bah*.

He notes that the word *"shanah"* is also the root word for "learning." He explains that if the sinner knows how to learn, he will attempt to justify his transgression and find a dispensation – *heter* – for his transgression. Thus, the passage would now read: Once a man has committed a transgression once, he learned and he devised a *heter* for his transgression. Permitted? How could that come into one's mind? Rather, in his own mind he perceives it is permitted.

The author of *Noam Elimelech*, R' Elimelech of Lizhensk, suggested that when one wants to correct a bad character trait he should reverse to the other extreme for a period of forty days.

< 62 >

Texting Addiction

< 63 >

Texting Addiction

The Mishnah in Pirkei Avos (3:1) states: "Consider three things and you will not come into the grip of sin: Know from where you came, where you are going, and before Whom you will give justification (din) and reckoning (v'cheshbon)."

The Vilna Gaon asks: What is the difference between "din" and "cheshbon"?

He explains that "din" (justification) refers to the Heavenly judgment one will confront with regard to his misdeeds and transgressions.

"Cheshbon" (reckoning) refers to the calculation that will be made in Heaven for all the good deeds, Torah learning and accomplishments one could have achieved during the time he transgressed.

< 65 >

Miriam's Story

Over the years I have found that teenagers, girls and boys alike, tend to eagerly embrace the new technology that is introduced to society at a dizzying pace. They seem to have an innate ability to master the electronics and are instantaneously proficient as well.

Miriam was a good student in high school, conscientious and studious. When she was in the twelfth grade, her parents finally capitulated and allowed her to get her own cell phone. Miriam was staying late for G.O. activities and play practice, and they preferred to be able to maintain contact with her when she traveled home alone on the train after rush hour. Miriam discovered that if she wanted to really keep in touch with her friends, she would be better off upgrading her phone so that she could have texting ability. She immediately did so, and discovered the wonderful world of SMS messaging.

Texting opened windows and doors to friends, and more friends. Her social circle burgeoned. Texting was captivating, appealing, and much more "cool" than just "talking" on the phone. You could reach anyone, at any time, in a moment's time. You could reach everyone, every time, no matter where you were. When Miriam got her driver's license, she couldn't wait to let EVERYONE know the good news. She had expanded her "group" contacts so that important news could be sent en masse to all her friends instantaneously. Miriam became very adept at texting; she could even text without looking at the keys.

At first it was just exciting to be able to communicate with everyone so effortlessly. Then it became a necessity; Miriam could not be without her phone for any given period of time. It was with her every waking moment. But then it took over her life. She was preoccupied with her phone, to the exclusion of any and all activities that required concentration,

< 66 >

focusing, or her undivided attention. Even her sleep was not impervious to the texting malady. She slept with the phone next to her so that she could hear any incoming messages as well as send her own message if she had something to say in the middle of the night. After a few months, even the Shabbos was no longer sacrosanct.

It didn't take long after that for the "disinhibition effect" to set in. Miriam found it extremely liberating to be able to "loosen up" and say whatever was on her mind. Although, she was by nature more reticent, she found it less intimidating to share her emotions and thoughts when texting. What was more disturbing was that she was equally uninhibited about publicizing her criticism, dislikes and aversions about people whenever she felt like it.

One evening at supper, she was texted: Did u no Michal is seeing s/o already on 4th date?

Some quick text networking informed Miriam that it was indeed serious and the guy was a great catch. Miriam did not share a good history with Michal. She had once been offended by Michal, and her long-buried antagonism and resentment came bubbling to the surface. Why did Michal have all the good luck, while she, Miriam, couldn't even get a date?

Miriam immediately typed a message, full of bitterness and rancor about Michal, sparing no detail of the long-ago incident in school. Her nimble fingers danced across the keys, fueled by her rage. When she sent the message, however, unbeknownst to her she inadvertently directed her message to her "group" of friends instead of responding to the sender alone. Needless to say, the repercussions rippled around the world as the *lashon hara* spread like wildfire to all of Miriam's three hundred and some "friends."

Miriam was inundated with sad telephone calls and

< 67 >

indignant texts from many of the recipients, who were not happy to be part of such unpleasantness. About two hours later Miriam received a call from Michal herself, the hapless victim of Miriam's addiction gone awry.

• • •

< 68 >

With the introduction of mobile phones, society moved into a new era. The advantages of the cell phone are numerous and indisputable. It is the drawbacks that are of concern, because as with many other indulgences in life, too much of a good thing often ends up being detrimental.

Technology quickly advanced, and cell phones didn't merely handle telephone calls; carriers offered SMS as an add-on feature. It became the norm when teens, in particular, adopted it as an alternate form of basic communication with their friends. Before long, everyone and their teenagers had a cell phone – of course with texting capability. Even parents who were wary of allowing an Internet connection, eventually yielded to teenagers' requests for texting ability on their phone.

Texting developed a language of its own. Those less experienced with the keyboard worked to perfect their skills, some using two thumbs, others using two alternate fingers. In no time, texting became more than a past-time; it became an obsession and an addiction.

Psychologists discuss many negative aspects of texting, but it is important to also be aware of the halachic and hashkafic ramifications.

< 69 >

Ben's Story

Ben, a 17-year-old young man, whom I had known for a few years, requested a meeting with me to discuss a painful situation in his life. Sensing the gravity of his concern I tried to accommodate him and agreed to meet him later in the evening.

As he sat down across my desk, he seemed slightly preoccupied and discomfited. He couldn't seem to make eye contact and kept averting his eyes downward. His hands seemed to be in a state of perpetual motion. I was actually taken aback by his manner and his apparent distraction, especially in light of the fact that it was he who had initiated the request to meet.

During the course of our conversation I received an important call and had to excuse myself to be able to speak in private. When I concluded the call, I walked back toward my office. As I reached the doorway of my office I saw that Ben had his cell phone in hand and was busily texting. I immediately understood what had been going on for the last hour. Ben had obviously been doing that the entire time that we had been talking.

Despite the fact that Ben was in dire need of all the help he could get, and it was critical that he pay close attention to the details of our discussion, he was nevertheless so absorbed in his compulsion to text, that he could not put aside his phone even during the time he was meeting with me.

• • •

< 70 >

Text messaging has become the preferred method of basic communication between teens and their friends, with more than two-thirds of teens more likely to use their cell phones to text their friends than to talk to them by cell phone. However, their preoccupation with this pastime in the company of others, at the dinner table, and while having a conversation is both offensive and disrespectful. Parents, teachers, friends, acquaintances, as well as the bank teller, the clerk in the store, and the waiter are sacrificed at the altar of the texters.

HaGaon HaRav Eliyahu Dessler (1892-1953) writes that *middos tovos* (good character traits) are precious commodities. One must cultivate his character, preserve his qualities, and correct those behaviors that need improvement. Our character traits are the tools we work with to elevate our spiritual level and prepare our share in the World-to-Come.

The Talmud *(Berachos 28b)* teaches us that when R' Eliezer fell ill his disciples visited him and asked him for advice on how they could secure their share in the World-to-Come. He said to them: "Be considerate of the honor of your colleagues ..."

The Darkei HaShleimus refers to the prayer of *"Yotzer Ohr* – Who forms light" and cites the Avos D'Rebbe Nosson on the words, "The angels in Heaven all accept upon themselves the yoke of Heavenly sovereignty from one another, and grant permission to one another to sanctify the One Who formed them ..." He notes that when the angels in Heaven begin to say *shirah* – sing praise to the Al-mighty – each one says to the other, "You begin first because you're greater than I am."

We learn from here that even when a person is engaged in performing *mitzvos*, it is nevertheless forbidden to offend another person and one must follow the guidelines of *derech eretz*.

It is interesting to observe that often when people need to

< 71 >

discuss something sensitive or emotional they avoid looking at the other person and will keep their eyes averted. Texting allows a similar process. It allows people to articulate thoughts and feelings they would never say face-to-face. The words can, thus, be malicious, hurtful and critical.

When an individual uses his text communication ability to promulgate derogatory information, or spread a rumor about an individual with his texting, one transgresses many prohibitions – *rechilus* (tale-bearing), *sheker* (falsehood), *ona'as devarim* (causing pain with words), *sinas chinam* (baseless hatred), *tzediyas rei'a* (entrapping a neighbor) and more.

The Chofetz Chaim lists 31 *mitzvos* which may be transgressed when one speaks or listens to *lashon hara*. He notes in his *Sefer Shemiras HaLashon* that the prohibition of *lo selech rachil* (you shall not be a gossipmonger) includes publicizing something negative by any means of communication, not only through speech – i.e., newspapers, circulars, and texting *(Hilchos Lashon Hara 1:8)*. Even if every detail of the information is accurate it still constitutes *rechilus*, and one transgresses an *issur d'oraysa*, a Torah prohibition. If there is any untruth in the information then one transgresses the *issur* (prohibition) of *motzi shem ra* (slander).

The Ramchal explains that any speech that results in the harm of an individual in Klal Yisrael, whether it is instigated face to face or behind his back, is considered *lashon hara*. This sin is despised by Hashem, and it is considered as if one has denied the existence of Hashem. Thus, if one embarrasses another person, he is not only punished for the ultimate shame he caused, but he is also liable for the terrible sin of *lashon hara*.

Our sages further discuss the Talmud *(Bava Metzia 58b)* which states, "One who embarrasses his friend in public it is as if he has killed him." Although the Torah did not include this prohibition within the category of speaking *lashon hara*,

< 72 >

nevertheless, that does not grant one the liberty to engage in the practice of insulting and shaming another person.

The Tiferes Yisroel writes that one who spreads *lashon hara* or *rechilus* about a person – a being created by Hashem personally, in fact diminishes Hashem's Name and causes the greatest *chilul Hashem* (desecration of Hashem's Name).

The Talmud *(Kiddushin 66a)* relates a fascinating story about Yannai HaMelech (103 BCE – 76 BCE) who waged war in Kuchlis and was victorious. Upon his return he made a victory celebration and invited all the *chachmei Yisrael* (Torah sages).

One person, Elazar ben Po'irah, was jealous of the *chachamim*, and he told the King that the *chachamim* opposed his reign.

"What shall I do?" the king asked Elazar.

Elazar advised the king to appear before the *chachamim* with the *tzitz* on his forehead.

Yannai did so, and one of the *chachamim* there said, "Let the crown of kingdom suffice for you. Leave the *kehunah* to the descendants of Aharon."

The Braisa notes that, in truth, Yannai was a descendant of Aharon, but there was a rumor that his mother had been captured in the city of Modi'in and dishonored. The law is that a wife who has been captured is invalidated from the *kehunah*, and her children cannot serve as *Kohanim*.

The rumor was not confirmed, but the harm was done. The *chachamim* departed in anger because of the false accusation.

Elazar ben Po'irah then said, "That is the law for even the most humble man in Yisrael. You are a king and a *Kohen*, should

< 73 >

that be your law too?"

Elazar then advised him to kill all the *chachamim*.

"But what about the Torah?" asked Yannai HaMelech.

"The Torah is rolled up and lying in the corner; whoever wants can come and learn from it."

Yannai HaMelech killed all the *chachamim* and indeed the world was desolate until Shimon ben Shetach came (120 – 40 BCE) and restored the Torah to its former glory.

Chazal tell us that *tzora'as* (leprosy) is a Divine punishment for the sin of *lashon hara*. The *Sefer HaKaneh* states that nowadays instead of *tzora'as* we have the suffering of poverty.

Many people think that rumors are innocuous and innocent. In truth, being a link in the continuation of a rumor may be aiding and abetting a murder.

Rumors that cause embarrassment to an individual, or a group of people, fall under the category of shaming a face in public. It is considered as if the person has spilled blood, and he does not have a *chelek* in *olam haba*, a portion in the World-to-Come.

If one engages in the dissemination of rumors, or is on the receiving end and believes the rumors, he transgresses "*Midvar sheker tirchak* – Distance yourself from falsehood," violating an *issur d'oraysa*.

The *mefarshim* explain that the Torah uses the word *tirchak* (distance), as opposed to *tishmor* (guard yourself), to highlight the importance of disassociating oneself from any trace of *sheker*, falsehood. Often times, in an effort to lend more veracity to the rumor, it will be embellished with some truth.

< 74 >

The Zohar tells us in *Parshas Pekudei* that when one spreads a rumor, or any forbidden speech, he impedes his *tefillos* and *bakashos* (requests) from rising upwards. There are adversaries whose task it is to seize any falsehoods, untruths or forbidden words that a person utters. Then, later, when that individual speaks holy words of *tefillah* they become defiled. The strength of their holiness is weakened and they are not meritorious.

The ease with which one can communicate by texting dominates our lives, detracting from our focus in all areas of concentration. People are texting while walking with their baby carriages, while crossing the street, while driving their cars – often resulting in physical harm to themselves and others. Teenagers are busily corresponding while in class and in *shiur.*

A very sad and disturbing development is the proliferation of texting in *shul*, even during *tefillah*, that threatens the spiritual wellbeing of its users.

A close colleague of mine related the following incident to me:

During *krias haTorah* (the reading of the Torah) the *gabbai* called out the name of an individual for an *aliyah*. He happened to be sitting in the back looking down, as if immersed in learning and didn't respond to his name. The *gabbai* called out his name once again, this time a little louder. The man still did not respond. The *gabbai* could not imagine why he hadn't heard, so he approached the individual. By that time, of course, the entire congregation was curiously following the proceedings. When the *gabbai* tapped him on the shoulder, the person looked up and turned red with embarrassment. He had been so engrossed in his texting that he had not realized that his name had been called three times to come up to the Torah.

Individuals are so conditioned to respond to the buzz on their phone indicating an incoming message, they are addicted.

< 75 >

They often feel that since texting is not verbal communication it does not constitute an interruption, or *hefsek,* during prayer and they do not turn off their phones when they are in *shul.*

HaRav Dessler notes that the essence of *tefillah* is the *kavanah,* which arouses the core element of purity in one's heart. It is very difficult for one who prays without *kavanah* to be meritorious, although he is still obligated to pray so that he should not forget that duty. He states that much of the Divine Assistance that one needs in life is dependent on his *kavanah* when he prays.

The Lev Eliyahu writes in a similar vein and refers to the Rambam who defines a *korban* as an expression of *hiskarvus* (advancing closer). *Tefillah* today replaces the *korbanos* of the *Beis HaMikdash* and affords us the opportunity of drawing nearer to Hashem. The Lev Eliyahu cites the *pasuk (Shemos 23:25),* "You shall worship Hashem and He shall bless your bread and your water ..." and explains that many serve Hashem, but Hashem scrutinizes the *tefillos* to determine the sincerity of each one's words as he prayed, and then blesses the sustenance of each individual accordingly. Thus, says the Lev Eliyahu, the response that one gets from Hashem is relative to the passion that he invests in his *tefillah.*

Parents, in particular, often maintain a false sense of security because their children do not have a phone with Internet capability. In fact, though, with texting on their cell phones they can be in touch with a network of people, many unfamiliar and unsavory.

< 76 >

Leah's Story

L eah went out with her friends on Motzoei Shabbos to one of the local eateries. It was one of the "in" places, noisy, full of people, with plenty of good food. The girls were there a couple of hours talking and eating, enjoying the evening and the time spent together. When they left, each of the girls paid her bill; Leah paid hers with a personal check.

When she got home, Leah noticed that she had a text message on her phone. She didn't recognize the number, and texted back, "Who are you?"

"Guess," was the response.

Her interest piqued, Leah kept texting. "Give me a hint."

"I'm a good friend of yours," appeared on the screen.

The interaction continued, although Leah still had no clue with whom she was communicating.

The texting sessions continued back and forth for about a week.

The following Shabbos night when Leah's phone buzzed, the message from her unknown "text pal" read, "Let's get together."

Imagine Leah's disbelief and shock when she discovered that she had been corresponding with the waiter at the café she had visited a week earlier. When Leah had paid with her check, the waiter had jotted down her phone number so that he could contact her.

< 77 >

When Leah complained to the manager, she was amazed at his indifference. "What? He did that again? You don't honestly expect me to regulate his conduct after hours."

• • •

< 78 >

Obviously the power of control is in our hands. We must control our impulsive behavior, our intense need to communicate with others – even if they are unknown to us – and our harmful habits and compulsions.

A disturbing new trend that has emerged especially among teenagers is the casual texting and exchange of inappropriate photos. Often when these messages are sent, or received, the only known is the phone number, not the person actually reading the message or keying in the text. What is more, these photos often wind up being seen by a much wider audience than ever intended, because the original recipient does have Internet capability, and he/she decides to upload those photos to Facebook to share with others. An impulsive whim to have some fun can suddenly become a humiliating experience that haunts one for years.

HaGaon HaRav Elchonon Wasserman presents a very interesting interpretation of the *pasuk (Bereishis 32:26)*, "The hip socket of Yaakov was dislocated as he [the angel of Eisav] wrestled with him."

He states that the "hip socket" symbolizes the *tinokos shel beis rabban* (children who learn Torah) who have been the essential foundation of our people for thousands of years. However, notes Rav Wasserman, even this foundation will become unstable during the *ikvesa d'meshicha* (era before the arrival of Mashiach) because of the assaults that will be launched from within and without.

Perhaps most alarming is the unprecedented progression of adolescents' compulsion to text, to the point where they can no longer set aside the cell phone for the holy day of Shabbos. Shabbos is one of the mainstays of the Torah and Judaism. The integrity of Judaism is based on *shemiras* Shabbos (the guarding of the Shabbos) and throughout our history of inquisitions, pogroms, the Holocaust, and the gulags, Jews old and young

< 79 >

alike self-sacrificed to observe the sanctity of Shabbos. Now the honor of Klal Yisrael is being attacked at its very core.

Ordinarily, the *yetzer* (the Evil Inclination) would never be able to prevail upon us to profane the Shabbos. Who among us would ever consider writing on Shabbos or driving on Shabbos? Would we ever think of consciously doing any of the 39 *melachos* (categories of labor that are prohibited on Shabbos)?

However, texting has become an uncontrollable habit, and the *yetzer* has cleverly harnessed this addiction in its war against *shemiras* Shabbos and its assault on the sanctity of Shabbos. The intent of the *yetzer* is to exploit texting as the initial action that will *chas v'shalom* (G-d forbid) set in motion a domino effect of full *chilul* Shabbos (desecration of the Shabbos). This could be compared to one who mistakenly eats something on a fast day and then feels he might as well continue eating since he has already broken his fast.

The Michtav M'Eliyahu notes that Shabbos is a creation of its own; it is a world of rest. This does not connote a sense of lethargy or indolence, but rather a respite from the material pursuits of the world. This reprieve for the soul is the essence of a life of spirituality.

The *Medrash Bereishis* relates that when Kayin came away from his judgment for having killed Hevel he encountered Adam HaRishon.

Adam HaRishon quered, "What was your verdict?"

Kayin replied, "I did *teshuvah* and I made a compromise."

Adam struck his face and exclaimed, "Such is the power of *teshuvah* and I didn't realize it!"

He immediately rose and said the psalm *Mizmor Shir L'Yom*

< 80 >

HaShabbos (Tehillim 92) to express his great joy for the gift of repentance.

HaGaon HaRav Michel Yehuda Lefkowitz asserts that we learn from here that Shabbos is a day of *teshuvah* from which is derived the *kedushah* (holiness) of the Shabbos day. The Talmud *(Pesachim 54a)* states that *teshuvah* is one of the seven things that was brought into existence before the world was created, because without the capacity for repentance the world would not be able to endure. One who observes Shabbos as a channel to elevate himself spiritually and to be inspired to achieve the loftiness of *teshuvah* merits to have the *kedushah* of Shabbos rest upon him.

< 81 >

Help

Internet and texting addictions have very similar components. Although I have chosen to address the halachic and hashkafic aspects of texting that are problematic in a separate chapter, the indications of addiction as well as the necessary therapeutic assistance are very similar.

For those caught in the Shabbos texting conundrum, I can offer the following additional suggestions:

- If you find you are texting excessively, without control, it would obviously be too difficult to apply the brakes just in time for Shabbos. In order to try to refrain from texting on Shabbos, begin to rein in your texting during the week.

- Give away your cell phone to a responsible individual for Shabbos. Of late I have become the keeper of a number of cell phones for young people over Shabbos and Yom Tov.

- Learn a *sefer* or a book that deals with the holiness of Shabbos. Having a more comprehensive understanding of the 39 *melachos* will help clarify the prohibition of texting on Shabbos.

- Make plans for Shabbos that will keep you busy so that you are not overcome by boredom.

- If you feel the texting has gotten out of hand, or there is an element of OCD, seek proper help.

< 82 >

Drug Addiction

< 83 >

Drug Addiction

A man who was alleged to have committed a crime was put in prison until his day in court. Judgment day arrived and the prisoner was escorted to the courthouse by one of the guards. In order to ensure that the prisoner could not escape, the guard handcuffed himself to the convict and together they walked through the streets to the courthouse.

*People in the street gathered to jeer and boo as the detainee was led on his way. Defensively, he called out, "You're mistaken. He's not taking **me**; I am the one who is taking **him** to the judge. I put **him** in handcuffs."*

The group fell silent for a moment, and then one wise guy in the crowd shouted, "If that's true, so open the handcuff on your hand. If you can free yourself that will prove that you control him. Otherwise, it will be confirmed that he has power over you."

The Alter of Navardok tells us that if one wants to determine whether he has become completely entrenched in a difficult situation he should ascertain whether he can get out of his predicament by himself.

The psalmist writes (Tehillim 130), "From the depths I called You, Hashem."

The Malbim comments on the plural form of "depths" and notes that man can find himself in the depths of despair either physically or spiritually. An addiction indeed affects the individual in this manner; it has the ability to break the body and the soul. With siyata d'shmaya (Divine Assistance) he will be able to break free and start anew, as the psalmist concludes, "And He shall redeem Israel from all its iniquities."

< 85 >

Alex's Story

A number of years ago I found myself unexpectedly in a Virginia hospital waiting room on a Friday afternoon in the summer. Knowing that I had a long wait ahead of me, I decided to check out the clergy registry and visit some of the Jewish patients. There were five Jewish names on the list. I chose to visit the patient on the thirteenth floor.

When I exited the elevator, I noticed that the corridor was entirely deserted and eerily quiet. Room 1349 was all the way at the other end. I knocked on the closed door, but no one answered. I knocked again and still no one answered. Fearing that perhaps the patient was too ill or feeble to call out, I opened the door.

When I entered, Alex lay with his back to the door. He turned slowly and I was saddened to see a young sickly-looking man of about eighteen, with a drawn face, whose skin was pallid and gray.

He looked at me suspiciously. "Who are you? What do you want?" he questioned belligerently.

I explained that I was a rabbi. I had seen his name on the clergy registry, I said, and had come to see how he was feeling.

"Who sent you? Did the social services agency tell you to come? Did my mother call you?" He seemed very agitated.

I explained again patiently, in a soothing voice, "No one sent me. I only came to visit a fellow Jew. When I saw your name I knew you were Jewish so I came up to visit you."

Alex put his head in his hands and began crying bitterly, all the while saying, "Nobody sent you. Nobody sent you."

< 86 >

After two minutes he stopped crying and said, "It was very nice of you to come and see me, a stranger. It was nice." He seemed to relax a bit.

"Alex," I said, "why are you here?"

He began to answer in half-sentences. Haltingly, and bit by bit, his tragic history unfolded. As he spoke, almost as if against his will, years of pent-up thoughts and emotions began pouring out in a torrent.

"I've been here for three months. I'm not really sick, you know. I guess you could say I am – I'm sick in the head. I'm sick in my heart. I'm sick of everything."

He stopped for a moment. "I'm here three months ... do you know why, Rabbi? Not for the usual reasons." He paused again, as if he could not bear to say it, "I am ... was ... a drug addict. A drug addict," he said again bitterly. "Now I'm clean, but who knows?

"I started doing drugs when I was only fourteen, for no reason. I had a regular childhood, but a lot of the other kids were doing it. I was curious, and I wanted to try it. Then you know what happens. I tried it once, twice, three times, and I was hooked. I began to act weird. I lied; I stole. In the beginning my parents had no idea why I was acting so crazy. They tried talking to me, to my teachers, to the school counselors. Nothing helped. I just kept on doing things my way. I couldn't stop. It took quite a while for my parents to catch on.

"When they found out, my parents tried to help me. I admit it – they tried to help me. But I didn't want to be helped. I just wouldn't stop. I couldn't stop. I left home when I was sixteen and roamed the streets. It's an awful story – you've probably heard it before, Rabbi.

< 87 >

"When even I couldn't stand myself anymore, I came to the rehabilitation center, the detox program in the hospital.

"While I was on the street I kept in touch with my parents from time to time. I would call them, mostly to ask for money. Then I called to tell them I was in the hospital. But in all these months they haven't once come to see me. Recently I let them know I was being released soon. You know what they told me? They said, 'Don't bother coming home. Your stuff is out on the street.'"

Alex began to cry again, hard and uncontrollably. "I don't blame them. I have no place to go from here. Who knows where I'll be three months from now? Probably right back where I was before. Sometimes I think I should just ... you know ... kill myself. I think it would be best for everyone. I'm scared, Rabbi.

"I've gotta tell you, I'm really scared. I don't want to go back to the way I was. I want to change. I want to turn my life around, but I don't know how. I don't know where to start.

"You're the first person who ever showed he cared about me – not because I'm your patient, or your kid or something – but just because I am a human being."

Alex stopped talking and I thought he had finished. Then he added, "And a Jew. You'll never know how much I appreciate that."

At that moment the words of the Rashi I had been learning earlier in the day *(Devarim 21:7)* sprang to mind: "Our hands did not spill this blood." (When an unidentified body is found on the road between two cities, the citizens of each city must come together and say that the person did not die because they had allowed him to leave their city unaccompanied.) Unfortunately, no one would accompany Alex. He would leave the hospital all alone, with no one to help him along the difficult road ahead.

< 88 >

The responsibility was ours.

I spoke to Alex as long as time would allow, encouraging him and offering him hope. I told him, '"Alex, you do have a purpose in life. You do have someone who cares about you. You are a Jew. You have a beautiful heritage, and a birthright. Most importantly, you have Hashem, Who loves each and every one of His children and cares deeply about each one."

We spoke a while longer, and then I wished Alex a good Shabbos. As I headed towards the door, he asked very tentatively, "Rabbi, will you come again?"

I assured him that I definitely would.

That Shabbos I could not stop thinking about Alex's situation. I kept thinking about this floundering *neshamah* desperate to be rescued. He was a Jew who felt so alone in the world yet was unaware of how close his solace actually was.

Motzoei Shabbos, as soon as I had made *Havdalah*, I returned to the hospital and spoke with Alex late into the night.

Every day for the next two weeks I visited Alex. We spent many hours in philosophical discussion, touching on numerous areas of Yiddishkeit, Torah, hashkafah and halacha. I also mentioned that it would be important for him to have an opportunity to be introduced to Jewish learning and casually suggested the idea of learning in a special yeshiva for people with little or no background.

The day of Alex's release, I came to the hospital one more time. I found Alex out of bed, pacing the room impatiently. His physical appearance was much improved, compared to the first time I had seen him. But more importantly, I saw a certain measure of serenity, even a bit of self-confidence, that had not been there before.

< 89 >

Alex excitedly shook my hand, and we sat down to talk. I knew this would be our last meeting. We spoke a while – about life, about *emunah*, and about Alex. I then gave Alex a *bracha* and wished him continued *hatzlacha* as he made his way down the long path to complete recovery.

As I rose to leave, Alex jumped up from his chair and said, "Rabbi, wait!" I stopped.

"I've been thinking. I've really been thinking All my life I've been looking for something, some crutch, to help me through. I needed outside things to make me feel good. Until now it was drugs." He gave a bitter laugh. "Yeah, I felt good, but it only lasted for a little while. Rabbi, tell me the truth. Do you think they would take me?"

"Who, Alex? Do I think who would take you?"

"Do you think that yeshiva you mentioned for guys like me – I don't know the first thing about Judaism; I didn't even have a *bar mitzvah* – do you think they would accept me?"

Alex was looking at me expectantly. It was the first glimmer of hope I had seen in his eyes since I had first met him.

I said reassuringly and emphatically, "Alex, I don't **think** they will take you; I **know** they will."

It was time for me to return to New York, and I made sure to elicit a promise from Alex that he would maintain contact with me. For the first few weeks after his discharge, Alex would call about once a week. He was having a difficult time adjusting to a "normal" life, relying on the charity of a secular organization and with no familial affections. I became concerned about his ability to stay clean on his own without a strong support system, so I encouraged him to come up to New York. I wanted to make sure that his recovery was not

< 90 >

sabotaged in any way before the *z'man* (new school term) began at the yeshiva we had discussed.

He seemed amenable to my suggestion over the phone, and I wired him the money to come to New York.

That was the last I heard from Alex. Sometimes, when a homeless derelict hustles me for a handout I peer into his face, looking for Alex. I think about him often and wonder about his fate.

• • •

< 91 >

Drug addiction is a chronic complex disease of compulsive drug use. The drug of choice varies, and runs the gamut from marijuana to cocaine, steroids, inhalants, and prescription drugs that include barbiturates, stimulants, hallucinogens and pain relievers. While each drug produces different physical effects, repeated use of any and all of them causes changes in the brain that perpetuate the cycle of drug abuse.

People experiment with drugs for many different reasons. Many first try drugs to have a good time, to be able to study better, to lose weight, because of peer pressure, to relieve depression or stress, to improve athletic performance, or out of simple curiosity.

The Rambam wrote the *Hanhagos HaBriyos* in 1198. The Sultan of Egypt, who was ill from physical ailments and also suffered from depression, asked the Rambam for medical advice. In his *sefer* the Rambam talks about good health care, exercise, diet, general hygiene, not engaging in unhealthy lifestyles, and being very careful to keep away from anything that harms the body.

We receive guidance from the Torah that all matters pertaining to human life and health should be carefully assessed. The Rambam states *(Hilchos Rotzei'ach 11:4)* that refraining from at-risk activity is derived from the *pasuk*, "*Hishamer lecha u'shmor nafshecha me'od* – guard yourself and guard your soul."

Drug use does not automatically lead to drug abuse. Moreover, the exact cause of drug abuse and dependence is not known. It is known that there are certain factors that may make one vulnerable to become addicted to drugs, such as:

- Easy access to drugs
- Low self-esteem or problems with relationships
- Abuse, neglect, or other traumatic childhood experiences

< 92 >

- Depression or anxiety disorders
- Environmental stress
- Peer pressure

The Talmud *(Berachos 32b)* relates the story of a righteous person who stopped to pray along the road. An officer approached him and greeted him, but the man did not respond.

The officer stood and waited until the conclusion of his prayers, and then exclaimed: You fool! Doesn't the Torah say *(Devarim 4:9)*, *"Rak hishamer lecha ushmor nafshecha me'od –* only take heed for yourself and take great heed for your soul" and *(Devarim 4:15)* *"V'nishmartem me'od l'nafshoseichem –* you shall greatly beware for your souls"? Why did you not reply when I greeted you earlier? If I had cut your head off with my sword who would have demanded from me satisfaction for your life?

The Talmud records the response of the righteous person who compared the act of prayer before Hashem to one who stands in front of an earthly king. "If you friend had come and given you greeting, would you respond?" asked the righteous man.

"No," replied the officer.

"And if you had responded what would they have done to you?"

"They would have cut my head off with a sword," replied the officer.

"If so," said the righteous man, "all the more when one stands in front of the King of kings he will not interrupt his prayers to return a greeting."

The Ksav Sofer notes that this narrative supports the principle that one must not only protect himself from external

< 93 >

danger, but he must also be very careful to guard his personal health and wellbeing,

There is also the rabbinic injunction against *chovel b'atzmo* – injuring oneself without a valid reason. In this context, one who sets himself in harm's way, i.e., puts himself in physical or mortal danger, is culpable for his oversight.

In his *Igros Moshe (Yoreh Dei'ah 3:35)* HaGaon HaRav Moshe Feinstein discusses the increased use of drugs and cites a number of reasons to prohibit it.

A person is commanded to guard his body (e.g. his health) as it says *(Devarim 4:15)* "*V'nishmartem me'od l'nafshoseichem.*" Drugs essentially harm and eventually destroy the body of a person.

Although some may argue *shomer pesayim Hashem* (Hashem protects the simple), R' Moshe writes in another context (*Igros Moshe, Choshen Mishpat 2:76*) that this principle only applies when two specific conditions are met: (1) the risks of the activity are indeterminable and (2) most people are willing to take a chance and engage in that pursuit. However the risks for drug users are clearly defined, especially as the habit escalates into a ruinous addiction. Moreover, although drug use has been steadily increasing, most of the rise is attributed to use among teenagers. This is especially alarming, as statistics indicate that the probability of addiction increases among those who start young and are daily users. In addition, although drug use is definitely more prevalent, it is clearly not in the category of *davar shedashu bo rabbim* (the masses are accustomed to it).

The Torah requires one to be grounded and aware of his actions at the time he executes *mitzvos*. Drugs have a mind-altering effect, interfering with one's ability to properly study Torah or fulfill the *mitzvos*.

< 94 >

The Torah *(Devarim 21:18-21)* speaks about the *ben sorer umoreh* (the rebellious son). The Talmud *(Sanhedrin 70a)* describes the *ben sorer umoreh* as a gluttonous young man who has specifically eaten meat and drunk wine in excess. Furthermore, he must have stolen money from his parents in order to purchase this meat and wine, and he must have consumed it in the company of deadbeats.

Alcoholism and drug addiction present a particular danger for teenagers. It is interesting to note, as well, that the Talmud highlights the company this young man keeps as a condition of his transgression. One of the strongest influences on youths is the peer pressure of their friends.

Upon his first offense the *ben sorer umoreh* is punished with lashes for stealing. If he continues his rebellious ways, he is executed by stoning despite the fact that he has not committed any major crime. Our sages tell us that this punishment was prescribed because of his anticipated delinquency in the future. In due course, he will become addicted to his eating habits and the need for alcohol and will eventually have to resort to robbing strangers of their money in order to feed his dependency.

R' Moshe notes that the *ben sorer umoreh* indulges excessively in food, which one needs for survival, and yet if he is consumed by his obsession it becomes an *aveirah*. Drug use is often motivated by a simple feckless pursuit of pleasure and a desire to feel good. Once one becomes a habitual user he resorts to criminal behavior as he is compelled to find ways to support his addiction that totally engulfs him.

R' Moshe also points out that parents of drug users suffer great anguish, and it is forbidden to cause one's parents unnecessary pain.

R' Moshe concludes with a strong warning against recreational drug use and urges every individual to make every

< 95 >

effort to prevent the proliferation of this disease which results in the transgression of the most severe Torah prohibitions.

Exclusive of nicotine and alcohol, marijuana is the most commonly abused illegal drug according to the National Institute on Drug Abuse.

The use of marijuana produces a sense of relaxation and heightened awareness of the visual, auditory and taste senses. However, extended use causes adverse effects such as paranoia, slowed thinking and reaction time, decreased coordination, increased blood pressure and heart rate, and learning and memory impairment. Since teens' brain systems are still maturing, marijuana use by teens adversely affects their development.

- In 2008, an estimated 2.2 million Americans used marijuana for the first time, more than half of them were under the age of 18.

- In 2009, a U.S. survey by the Substance Abuse and Mental Health Services Administration found that more than 2.6 million people, ages 12 and over, said that they were dependent on marijuana and/or hashish, a concentrated form of marijuana.

- In 2010, 21.4% of high school seniors had used marijuana in the past 30 days, while 19.2% smoked cigarettes

- By the time they graduate from high school, about 42% of teens will have tried marijuana.

< 96 >

Josh's Story

During a seminar at which I was one of the presenters, a young man seated close to the podium abruptly slumped over in his chair and fell to the floor, amid cries of shock and alarm from those seated around him.

I immediately identified the fallen man as Josh, someone who frequently attended my lectures, lying prostrate at the feet of his horrified wife, Marilyn. As I rushed toward them, amateur diagnoses – like a heart attack or an aneurysm – flashed through my mind.

By the time I reached them, I was relieved to see that Josh appeared to be coming around. His wife assured concerned onlookers that Josh was simply exhausted from working a double shift on extremely little sleep. The explanation seemed plausible enough and everyone, including myself, began to relax. After a few tense moments, the lectures resumed. The crisis had passed.

The incident had taken me by surprise, but I didn't give it much thought. I had known Josh and Marilyn for three years. In fact, I had officiated at their wedding. They were bright, well-educated, appeared to lack nothing; nor was I aware of any health problems. I did recall, though, that Josh had seemed somewhat distant and withdrawn the last few times we had met.

One can only imagine my shock when I received a frantic call from Marilyn, a few months later, informing me that Josh had been missing for almost two days! I listened carefully as she filled me in on the details of his disappearance.

"I thought he was just late returning from work, so I went to sleep, thinking he would surely arrive home soon. When I awoke the next morning, I realized that he had never come

< 97 >

home! I'm frantic! Tonight will be the second night Josh is missing, and I still have not heard from him! Please help me! I just don't know what to do!"

I desperately wanted to help the tearful woman find her husband, yet I felt as though part of the story was missing. The unusual circumstances of Josh's disappearance set off alarm bells in my head, and I asked Marilyn if there was any more information that she could possibly offer regarding Josh's strange disappearance.

"Oh, Rabbi," she cried. "I don't know how to tell you this! Josh sometimes has trouble coping with some of the everyday pressures at home and at work. He tried to find an easy escape, and he began experimenting with various drugs. He only meant to use them to relax a little bit, but before he knew it, he was hooked."

When I heard this shocking revelation, I felt personally responsible. Why couldn't they have confided in me? Why had I not been able to recognize the signs of substance abuse? Yet I knew that often people become experts at masking their deepest problems, whether it's substance abuse, physical and emotional abuse, eating disorders, or a myriad of other troubles.

The immediate concern at hand, however, was locating Josh. If, *chas v'shalom*, a child is missing there are wonderful organizations such as "Child Find" that are called in to help. Whom does one contact to track down a grown man who has vanished? The police had already been notified, the community was informed to be on the lookout, and several groups were organized to help comb the New York city streets in search of Josh.

I dedicated myself completely to the search efforts. It was difficult for me to undertake anything else during this period. Troubling thoughts raced through my mind as to what might

< 98 >

have happened – amnesia, overdose, or a drug deal gone sour. The possibilities were endless and not very optimistic.

Four days passed and, much to everyone's dismay, not a single lead surfaced regarding Josh's whereabouts. With each passing hour, the chances of finding him safe and sound grew more remote. I contacted various individuals, groups and organizations to pray on Josh's behalf. The search efforts intensified and flyers were printed with a description of Josh and a telephone number for anyone with information to call. On the bottom of every flyer there was even a reminder to pray for Josh's safe return. These flyers were distributed far and wide with many of them plastered on lampposts and bulletin boards throughout the city.

Four more agonizing days passed without a sign of Josh. He had been missing for over a week and some people despaired of ever seeing him again. It was close to midnight on Tuesday evening when my phone rang. As soon as I picked up the receiver, Marilyn, almost incoherent, shouted, "Josh called!! We know where he is! We're going to pick him up right now.'

I'll never forget that call. The prayers of the entire community had been answered. Josh was alive, on his way home! The next call I received was from an extremely soft-spoken Josh, thanking me for being there for him. It wasn't until the following day, though, that he revealed his incredible story to me.

He explained how his drug habit had begun as a seemingly harmless way to take his mind off his worries. But the narcotics quickly tightened their grip on him until he was no longer in control. He abhorred the reality that an ever-increasing segment of his days was consumed by drug use. He became despondent and disillusioned and eventually felt too ashamed of his addiction to remain in the community. He felt like he had failed his family, his acquaintances, and his friends. Soon his

< 99 >

pain became too agonizing to bear, and he decided to run away.

Life on the streets, though, was a dismal blur of drugs and depression. Josh had been wandering the streets of Manhattan that Tuesday night when he spotted a flyer on a lamppost. Upon closer inspection, he realized that the flyer depicted none other than himself. He was stunned that so many people were praying for him and it sent a powerful and encouraging message to Josh – that he was worthy of people's prayers. He felt renewed faith in himself.

Psychologists have long sought to discover why some people develop addictions. One theory is that addictions arise out of a need to correct an imbalance. Addicts become trapped, unaware and unable to deal with their thoughts, emotions and actions. They may drink, eat to excess, or as in Josh's case, take drugs, in order to disassociate themselves from their perceived deficiency. When Josh saw the flyer with its plea to pray on his behalf, he realized that many people truly **did** care for him. He understood that, even in his predicament, others still believed he was a worthwhile individual. He then understood, finally, that it was time to come home.

Josh had a long road to travel to wean himself from his dependency on drugs and to learn how to deal with his real life situations. He knew, though, that with a support group of people who really cared about him, he could do anything.

● ● ●

< 100 >

HaGaon HaRav Yosef Shalom Elyashiv discusses a similar situation, in his response to Rav Wosner concerning a woman who was apprehensive about her husband's drug abuse. Although he had made several attempts to achieve sobriety he had not been successful to date. As soon as he was stabilized, he would regress and disappear from home for lengthy periods of time. The woman was concerned that the time would come when her husband left home and did not return, leaving her an *agunah* (a woman whose husband has deserted her). She wanted her husband to appoint a *beis din* (rabbinic court) that could give her a *get* (divorce) on his behalf in the event that he did not return within a set period of time.

Prescription drugs are the second most commonly abused category of drugs, behind marijuana and ahead of cocaine, heroin, methamphetamine and other drugs. The National Institutes of Health estimates that nearly 20 percent of people in the United States have used prescription drugs for non-medical reasons.

Prescription drugs are appealing because of the feel-good experience they provide to the user. They are easier to obtain than street drugs. Prescription drugs are in the family's medicine chest, often even when they are no longer being used for their originally prescribed purpose. The availability of drugs from online pharmacies makes it almost effortless, even for minors, to buy the drugs without a prescription. Prescription drugs can also be bought on the street.

There is the misperception that prescription drugs are not as deleterious as illegal street drugs. In fact, serious health risks, including death, are associated with their abuse.

- In 2006 a total of 5.2 million people reported abuse of pain relievers.

- In 2007 a survey was conducted that found

< 101 >

prescription drug use had risen by 12% among young adults.

- According to a study by the Substance Abuse and Mental Health Services Administration, the number of teens and young adults (ages 12 to 25) who were new abusers of prescription painkillers grew from 400,000 in the mid-'80s to 2 million in 2000. A 50% increase in the abuse of tranquilizers was recorded between 1999 and 2000 alone.

- The National Institute on Drug Abuse's MTF Survey in 2010 found that about 1 in 12 high school seniors reported using Vicodin that was not prescribed for them, and 1 in 20 reported abusing Oxycontin.

One can develop an addiction to any of a number of prescription drugs that fall into three categories:

Painkillers, such as Vicodin, Oxycontin, Percocet and codeine, are powerful pain relievers that essentially reduce one's sense of pain and produce a sense of well-being and euphoria. If these narcotics and opioids are used for an extended period of time, a tolerance and physical dependency will develop. Effects of abuse include confusion, slowed breathing, drowsiness and sedation, and depression. "Cold turkey" withdrawal is extremely unpleasant.

Sedatives, or depressants, are used to treat sleep disorders, anxiety, or depression and slow down the central nervous system. Along with the sense of relaxation and well-being that is produced, these drugs tend to impair the user's ability to think clearly and react quickly. This category includes popular medications such as Valium, Xanax, and Librium. Effects of abuse include slurred speech, impaired coordination, confusion and disorientation, slowed breathing and decreased blood pressure, drowsiness and fatigue.

< 102 >

Ritalin and Adderall, often used to treat ADD/ADHD, and Dexedrine used to support weight loss, are stimulants, also known as uppers. These drugs speed up the central nervous system, producing increased energy that makes one feel less tired both physically and mentally. Their use over time, though, leads to paranoia, hallucinations, aggressive or impulsive behavior, sleep difficulties, and rapid or irregular heartbeat.

Other popularly abused drugs include hallucinogens, also known as psychedelics, that are mind-altering drugs, and inhalants such as common household solvents and gases, e.g. paint thinner, spray paint, and air fresheners.

When sniffed or inhaled, the chemicals found in inhalants giver the user a brief "high." However, the side effects include delusions and confusion and prolonged use can damage the brain. Overdosing is a very real risk, resulting in sudden heart failure.

Hallucinogens, such as LSD and Ecstasy, generate feelings of euphoria and heightened sensory awareness. Adversely, the user presents with an impaired perception of reality, increased heart rate and blood pressure, panic or paranoia, and tremors.

< 103 >

Elana's Story

Elana was a successful, fun-loving twelfth grader who attended an exclusive Jewish girls' school. She was intelligent, had many friends, loved a good time, and was looking forward to graduation at the end of the year. Elana had been accepted by one of the top colleges and had plans to study and prepare for a high-powered career.

One evening at the end of October, a number of girls gathered to celebrate the birthday of one of Elana's good friends. Elana did not personally know all of the teenagers there, but she was enjoying the evening immensely.

In middle of the party, Elana went into the kitchen for refills on ice, soda and salad. As she loaded the bowls of salad, one of the guests approached Elana and casually asked, "Hey, do you smoke?"

"No," said Elana.

"You never tried smoking? Are you serious?"

"No, I've never tried smoking," Elana answered hesitantly.

"Are you for real?"

"Yes. I've never actually understood the appeal of cigarettes. How about you?" asked Elana.

"Sure I smoke. Not all the time of course, just once in a while. But I'm not talking about cigarettes; I'm talking about the good stuff – weed!"

"Isn't that dangerous?" asked Elana. "Aren't you concerned about becoming addicted to it?"

< 104 >

"Not at all," the girl cavalierly reassured Elana. "Everybody does it. Nothing happens. You want to try some?"

"What? Here?"

"We could go out on the deck in the back if you'd like," said the girl.

"No," said Elana. "Someone will see us. I'd rather not."

"Fine. Let's go back and join the others."

Later that evening, as the party was drawing to a close, Elana bumped into the girl again. This time when she asked her if she would like to join her and have a "drag," Elana inexplicably said she would.

Although Elana didn't particularly enjoy her first experience with marijuana, the thought of tasting "forbidden fruit" was very exciting.

It was about two months later, and Elana had almost forgotten about the incident. The seniors were going on a mid-winter school trip to Washington and all the girls were paired up with roommates. Elana was surprised to see that her partner for the three-day trip was the girl she had met at her friend's birthday party.

The two girls actually got along very well and by the time the trip was over they had developed a strong friendship, which they maintained when they came back. Elana began to spend more time with her new friend, who introduced her to her own circle of very friendly girls from other schools in the area.

These girls would get together every weekend at someone's home to hang out. Elana enjoyed the camaraderie, although initially she did not join these girls in their drug escapades.

< 105 >

She did notice, though, that the drug of choice among the girls was not limited to marijuana. Ecstasy and cough syrup seemed popular, while some just enjoyed inhalants. Oddly enough, instead of being troubled by their conduct, Elana was almost envious. The girls were more relaxed. They were laid back and mellow – much less intense or driven than her usual friends at high school .

After a while, Elana yielded to temptation and tried a few tokes of marijuana again. She was pleasantly surprised to find that the experience was more enjoyable than the first time. She began to look forward to the weekly get-togethers for an opportunity to get a joint.

Then, as often happens, Elana began to progress to the use of "harder" drugs. Soon Elana was no longer experimenting with the easily available joints of marijuana and she needed more than the weekly pick-me-up. She began to associate with people who could provide her with the more potent drugs she craved.

Elana was always looking forward to her next fix. Most of her waking hours were spent obsessing about how she could get the drugs, from whom she could make the buy, and where she could get the money to pay for them. Making connections, getting high, coming down from her high – Elana was very busy. She would disappear from home for hours and offered flimsy excuses for her absences. Her attendance in school was erratic, and her grades began to suffer. Elana was no longer interested in her wardrobe or her appearance. Elana had become a "hopeless addict," in her own words.

The change was gradual but it was obvious that Elana was having serious problems. Finally, one day, one of her shifty dealers wandered into school looking to make a deal, and Elana was expelled from school.

< 106 >

Elana was so doped up that she was not interested in listening to anyone. Her parents pleaded and begged her to get help. The school administration reasoned with her. Her friends offered suggestions for rehab programs. All attempts to intercede were unsuccessful. Elana's plans and dreams for the future faded into oblivion.

On *Shivah Asar B'Tammuz* (the fast day of the 17th of *Tammuz*), Elana hit an all-time low. A few hours earlier Elana had hung loose at a "pharming party," with some new people she had met. Unfortunately, Elana had ingested a lethal combination of drugs and slipped into a coma. Thankfully, someone was with her and she was rushed to the hospital. It was touch-and-go for a while, but with Hashem's help Elana finally came through.

When she was finally released from the hospital, Elana went directly to a treatment facility for medically assisted detoxification. After three weeks, Elana could no longer be treated in an in-patient program. She was far from "cured" and needed serious help in many areas. She needed to be able to recognize and avoid situations that would trigger a relapse. She had to learn how to cope with her intense cravings for the drugs. It was a difficult struggle for Elana to reconnect with her old friends and break away from the druggies who had befriended her.

During the *Yamim Noraim* (High Holy Days), Elana was blessed with a spiritual awakening of sorts. The sparks of Yiddishkeit deep within her were fanned, and Elana was able to honestly assess the last few months of her unhealthy lifestyle. She recalled with fondness some old memories of her previous life and reevaluated her priorities and dreams for the future.

After much introspection, Elana made a conscious decision to do real *teshuvah* and to reclaim her soul. She made the necessary connections, dedicated herself to her studies as well as her rehabilitation, and established a strong support system.

< 107 >

Elana has been clean now for seven months. The healing process is arduous, but *baruch Hashem,* Elana continues to strive. She has enrolled in school, works for a few hours a week, and is committed to developing a closer relationship with Hashem. We who know her are greatly encouraged. We are all praying for her.

As Chazal tell us *(Shabbos 104a),* "*Ba litaher mesayim oso* – if one comes to purify himself he is helped."

• • •

< 108 >

In *Devarim (22:8)* we have the *mitzvah* of *ma'akeh:* "When you build a new house, you should make a fence for your roof, and you will not place blood in your house if someone falls from it."

Our sages tell us that one has the obligation to place a protective fence around any dangerous areas such as ditches and pits.

This *mitzvah* includes a *mitzvas aseh* (positive commandment) of building a fence, but there is also the *mitzvas lo sa'aseh* (prohibition) of "not to place blood in your house." Chazal tell us that this refers to more than simply building a literal physical fence or barrier around a dangerous roof. This commandment extends further and applies to any dangerous situation. For example, our sages tell us that it is a violation of Jewish law to drink from a polluted stream, or to put coins into one's mouth that may cause sickness from contamination. In effect, the law of *ma'akeh* requires the elimination of any possible danger or situation where people may be injured or hurt.

It is also noteworthy to mention the Torah dictum of *dina d'malchusa dina* – a concept that the laws of the country are binding on us. In our country, the laws prohibit the use of many different recreational drugs. Many prescription drugs that have been integrated for recreational use are heavily regulated by the government. Thus, if one is using these drugs illegally, or if one is in possession of certain drugs such as marijuana or cocaine, he is violating the law of the land.

< 109 >

Are You Addicted?

Drug abusers often try to keep their addiction a secret and/or to minimize any problems they may be experiencing. There are warning signs, however, that are troublesome and may indicate drug dependency.

- Does your craving for the drug take priority over all other aspects of your life, including family, friends, and career?

- Do you feel that you must have the drug in order to be able to deal with your problems?

- Has your drug use resulted in the elimination of many activities/hobbies you used to enjoy?

- Do you find that you need more of the drug in order to experience the same good feeling you used to enjoy with a lesser amount?

- Have you failed to quit your drug habit despite numerous attempts to do so?

- Do you continue to use drugs despite the adverse effects you are suffering?

- Do you find that you are completely preoccupied with concerns about how to acquire your drug supply?

- Do you find that a lot of your time is consumed recovering from the ill effects of the drugs?

- Are you stealing money, valuables or prescriptions in order to support your habit?

< 110 >

Help

Drug abuse and addiction is complex, and effective treatment must address a variety of issues. Overcoming addiction is not simply a matter of willpower, because extended use of drugs alters brain function and behavior, compelling the craving to use.

Initially, there is often a need for medically assisted detoxification to rid the body of drugs. Different chemical substances stay behind in the body longer than others. Moreover, just as each body reacts differently to the intake of drugs, similarly each body reacts differently to withdrawal from the addictive substance.

In order to facilitate a drug-free lifestyle, counseling is an important part of the recovery process to address:

- The psychological wellbeing of the addict

- Important lifestyle changes

- Ways of dealing with stress

- Development of productive and constructive functioning in the family, at work, and in society

Addicted individuals sometimes need medications to reduce their cravings for drugs and to allow them to achieve sustained abstinence.

Support, encouragement, comfort and guidance are essential components for addiction recovery. This includes:

- Family members

- Therapists and social workers

< 111 >

- Psychologists

- Clergy members

- Close friends

< 112 >

Spiritual Help

HaGaon HaRav Chaskel Levenstein (1895-1974) writes that when we are faced with *nisyonos* in this world, our task is to turn the darkness into light. He explains that the effort and labor that the person expends to overcome his challenges infuse him with great satisfaction. As a result, he is uplifted and encouraged. He will be able to discern the folly of a life of ersatz happiness and will embrace a type of life that is ideal, one that will allow him to experience true happiness. He will abandon his pursuit of a life of ephemeral enjoyment in exchange for an everlasting world of authentic happiness.

Since extended use of drugs alters the brain function and behavior, the drug addict perforce has a more difficult time with this *nisayon* in his *avodas Hashem*. Trapped in his addiction, unable to deal with his thoughts, emotions and actions, the drug addict is severely hampered. His senses are dulled, his memory and judgment abilities are impaired, and he is confused by either paranoiac or hallucinogenic thoughts. In effect, the drug addict's perception of reality is totally distorted. Yet, when the addict emerges from the darkness into the light he will indeed discover the joy of true contentment.

In the *Baruch She'amar* prayer we recite each morning, we deliver a series of praises and blessings of Hashem. Among them we mention, "Blessed is He Who redeems and rescues." HaGaon HaRav Avigdor Miller remarks that initially Hashem redeems the wrongdoer from his sin. However, just as a slave would not remain in his master's house once he has been liberated, similarly the sinner needs to be extricated from his place of danger, or his situation of misery. Accordingly, we pay tribute to Hashem, Who indeed redeems the sinner and then rescues him from his state of despair.

< 113 >

Alcohol Addiction

< 115 >

Alcohol Addiction

The Medrash relates that when Noach prepared to plant the vineyard, the Satan appeared and greeted him, "Shalom aleichem."

Noach responded in kind, "Aleichem shalom."

"What are you doing?" asked the Satan.

"I'm planting a vineyard," replied Noach.

"Why?"

"Because it's a good thing," said Noach. "We will have sweet fruit, and its juice will give us wine."

"If so," said the Satan, "perhaps we can be partners."

Noach agreed.

The Satan brought a lamb and slaughtered it. Then he brought a lion and slaughtered it. He also brought a monkey and a pig, which he slaughtered. Then he irrigated the plants with their blood.

Indeed, when one drinks the wine of the vineyard he partners with these animals, and his person becomes permeated with the animals' characteristics. Before a person partakes of drink he is like an innocent lamb. After he consumes a few drinks, he is emboldened like a lion. After he imbibes some more, a person acts like a monkey. He is loudmouthed and foul-mouthed, acting without dignity or self-respect. If he continues to drink, he appears like a pig, wallowing in his own vomit and filth.

< 117 >

Uri's Story

It was after 11:00 one icy winter night in *Shevat*, when I returned home from a series of lectures in Chicago. It was freezing cold and I looked forward to the warmth of my home and a hot meal. As I walked into the house, the study phone was ringing. Judging by the late hour, I suspected that the caller had an important *sheilah* (question of Jewish law).

In my rabbinic work over the years, I have received many *sheilos* (halachic questions) on every imaginable topic, especially concerning at-risk behaviors. That night's call was no different. Uri, a 23-year-old young man who lived out on the Island somewhere and attended my weekly *shiur,* wanted to meet with me to discuss something important. Since it was already late, we agreed to meet the following evening.

After the preliminary greetings, Uri explained that he needed some clarification about the laws of *kibbud av v'eim* – honoring one's parents. I outlined the parameters and then elaborated on various details. Unsure of what direction to take, I stopped for a moment and asked Uri specifically which point about *kibbud av v'eim* he was seeking to clarify.

"Well," said Uri, "if your father asks you to do something, do you always have to listen?"

I explained that performing a task for one's parent takes precedence most of the time. The exceptions would be if there was a timely *mitzvah* he must perform which no one else could do in his stead, or if the parent asks him to transgress a sin.

Uri did not seem satisfied with my answer, so I asked again, "What, in particular, did your father ask you to do that is bothering you?"

Uri looked miserable and squirmed uncomfortably in his

< 118 >

seat. Then he blurted out, "I believe my father has a drinking problem. When he comes home every evening from work he has a few glasses. Depending on the amount he imbibes, he may either get abusive and violent, or he may pass out on the couch. Shabbos has basically been ruined for the family. We've discontinued our practice of having guests a while ago. Often he doesn't even make it to *shul* on Shabbos morning because he's plastered. It's very embarrassing for us because, since there is only one *shul* in our neighborhood, everyone is aware that my father has not attended *shul* that morning. We make excuses – saying that he had to stay with his mother who is elderly and not well – but we're extremely uncomfortable. I'm sure people suspect the truth."

By now Uri had tears rolling down his cheeks, but I still didn't know what his *sheilah* was. "What is the question?" I gently inquired.

"My father has become very difficult and begun to shift many of his responsibilities to me. I pick up the groceries, service the car, call the insurance company ... Now my father has been asking me to pick up the liquor. Sometimes I tell him I forgot to run the errand and he gets very angry. He has threatened to ruin any opportunities I may have for *shidduchim* if I don't shape up and do his bidding."

Uri hung his head in embarrassment and said softly, "I know that he loves the bottle more than he loves his own children. My *sheilah* is, Rebbi, do I have to buy the whiskey for him?"

We discussed the situation in depth. There were a few considerations here, primarily the Torah prohibition of *lifnei iver lo siten michshol* (lit., you shall not place a stumbling block before the blind). Since excessive alcohol intake can be harmful and endangers the wellbeing of his family and others, I discussed with Uri the feasibility of somehow limiting his father's intake

< 119 >

and/or avoiding carrying out his father's wishes.

Uri had some difficulty with the suggestion and said he would discuss it with his younger brother, Ethan, and get back to me. Uri did call the next night to say that they would try to follow my recommendation, but he wasn't sure how it would work out.

Two weeks passed, and the liquor supply at home had run dry. Uri's father called him on his cell to stop by the liquor store on his way home from yeshiva and pick up a mixed case of gin, brandy and rum. With great *derech eretz*, Uri apologized that he would not be able to run that errand.

Uri's father was furious and angrily slammed the phone down. He then called Ethan. When Ethan got his father's call, he was in a dither. He recalled his agreement with Uri, but did not want to be the subject of his father's wrath. He rationalized that although the drinking was injurious to his father's health, many people engaged in behavior that was detrimental to their health. Moreover, his father's drinking was private at home, and perhaps preferable to carousing at the bars. Ethan also imagined that if he didn't run the errand, his father would probably find someone else to do his dirty work. With that calculation, Ethan complied and picked up the order at the liquor store.

After that I didn't hear from Uri, or his brother Ethan, for more than three months. When I did get their call, they were audibly upset and agitated and requested to meet with me as soon as possible.

I barely recognized the boys when I opened the door that evening. Uri and Ethan looked like they hadn't slept in days. I ushered them into my study to be seated, and then waited patiently to hear their story.

< 120 >

Uri began. "Two nights ago at 3:30 in the morning my mother knocked on my door to wake me up. It seems that, this time, my father left the house after his drinking binge, but he had still not returned. My father didn't usually stay out this late, and although my mother kept trying my father's cell phone her calls were automatically redirected to voice mail. She was now very concerned and wanted me to check out the bars in the area.

"Ethan and I drove out to a favorite haunt off the highway out of town, but he wasn't there. We then set off to systematically check out the other drinking holes we knew about. A few minutes later my cell phone rang. My mother was on the phone crying that she had received a call from the hospital that was forty minutes away. My father had been involved in a major automobile accident, totaling the car, and was in critical condition. He had been driving while intoxicated and was now undergoing emergency surgery.

"We swung by the house to pick up my mother and sped to the hospital. We sat for more than two hours before the surgeon came out to describe the severity of my father's injuries. He explained that the rescuers had to bring in the 'jaws of life' to extricate my father from the mangled car. He informed us that recovery would be long and arduous and he could not assure us that my father would heal completely."

I was horrified to hear the bleak prognosis offered by the doctor and as I sat there silently, absorbing the information they had just shared, Ethan cried out.

"That's not the worst of it! My *sheilah* is, if my father got drunk drinking from the bottles that I brought home for him, am I in any way halachically responsible for what happened?"

Postscript: Chacham Ovadia Yosef was asked to clarify the halacha in a situation where a child is requested to buy liquor for a parent who is an alcoholic. Chacham Yosef states

< 121 >

that one should not do this, because it endangers the parent's health and the parent may act in an embarrassing manner as a result of his drinking.

• • •

< 122 >

Alcoholism is a difficult word to say. How does it creep into one's life? Is it like a flu or a virus? Does one "catch" it?

Alcoholism, or alcohol dependence, is a negative pattern of alcohol use that leads to a number of problems. People who are addicted to alcohol need to drink alcohol in order to function normally and their drinking causes problems in their lives. The alcoholic's body actually depends on the alcohol. He has no control over whether he/she drinks. He also begins to build tolerance to the alcohol, requiring larger amounts of alcohol to achieve the desired effect, i.e. to get "high."

Psychologists have long sought to discover why some people develop addictions. One theory is that addictions develop to correct an imbalance. Alcoholics become trapped, unaware and unable to deal with their thoughts, emotions and actions. They need a crutch, or an escape, in order to disassociate themselves from their perceived deficiency, or a difficult moment in life. They use the alcohol to try to relieve anxiety, depression, tension, loneliness, self-doubt or unhappiness.

Sometimes it's peer pressure or simply a thrill-seeking adventure. A person takes one drink and another drink, and then a third. Before he knows it, he has exceeded the limit, and this may mark the beginning of the individual's decline.

Drinking alcohol makes people feel less inhibited and puts them at ease. It often helps break the ice in social gatherings, as it feels good to be doing what everybody else is doing.

Undoubtedly, drinking low amounts of alcohol increase the release of endorphins and produce an overall good feeling. In fact, moderate amounts drunk with meals may even be good for the heart and protect against certain types of strokes.

The Torah, in fact, states *(Tehillim 104:15)*, *"Yayin yesamach*

< 123 >

levav enosh – wine gladdens man's heart," and *(Mishlei 31:6)* "*Tenu sheichar le'oved v'yayin l'morei nofesh* – give strong drink to the anguished and wine to those of embittered soul."

However, drinking is like any other habit; it has to be engaged in with moderation. One cannot just drink indiscriminately. A woman who downs more than three drinks in a row, and a man who has more than four drinks on one occasion, are considered to be drinking in excess. One drink is either a 12-oz bottle of beer (4.5% alcohol), a 5-oz. glass of wine (12.9% alcohol), or 1.5 oz. of 80-proof distilled spirits. One must be careful when assessing his level of happiness or degree of depression. There are genetic differences in the response to alcohol and exceeding one's limit can actually trigger a desire for more.

We are commanded *(Vayikra 18:3)*, "*Uv'chukoseihem lo selechu* – and do not follow in their [Egypt's and Canaan's] traditions." Secular and religious holidays among non-Jews are often celebrated by limitless imbibing. Although our community should remain insular, at times we unfortunately pick up more practices from the outside world than we should. As a result, some have also embraced the practice of partaking in celebratory drinking, with negative consequences.

I often wonder what is accomplished by bringing a $300+ bottle of scotch to a *simcha* and showing friends and relatives how much one knows about the history or virtues of a particular bottle of whiskey. Years ago one bottle was brought out at a *simcha*, everyone made a *l'chaim* and truly rejoiced for the *baal simcha*. We must always remember that whatever values we emphasize, our children are observing and will incorporate those ideals into their lives. Drinking can be a learned behavior for which young people can acquire a strong taste, a liking for, and dependency.

It is hard to tell a person while he has the drink in his hand,

< 124 >

"I don't think you should have that." Usually the immediate response from that person is, "I'm old enough to know what I want, and I know it will not affect me."

Nor do people readily admit, "I've had one too many." The reason is because they are already ensnared in their own convoluted rationale and cannot be dissuaded in their inebriated state. Once they exceed their capacity for drink, the habit becomes like a huge wrecking ball in the hands of the *Satan* which can destroy the person himself and his family in one fell swoop.

The *pasuk* in *Mishlei (24:31)* states, "Do not look at wine becoming red, for to one who fixes his eyes on the goblet all paths are upright." The Talmud *(Yuma 75a)* explains that once a person is intoxicated, his judgment becomes impaired and "the entire world becomes to him like a plain," i.e. he sees no obstacles in order to attain that which he desires.

Countless examples are brought in the Torah and Talmud of the ruin that ensues excessive drinking.

In the Torah *(Bereishis 9:21* and *19:32)*, Noach's and Lot's drunkenness respectively resulted in tragic consequences.

In *Parshas Shemini* we read of the death of Aharon's two oldest sons, Nadav and Avihu. Our sages note that this chapter is immediately followed by the prohibition of *"shesuyei yayin,"* that a *kohen* may not perform the *avodah* under the influence of alcohol. The *Medrash Vayikra Rabbah* cites the view of R' Yishmoel that Nadav and Avihu were not in the proper spiritual frame of mind to enter the *Mishkan* for they had partaken of wine.

Similarly, we read *(Esther 1:10)*, "… when the heart of the king [Achashverosh] was merry with wine he told … to bring Queen Vashti before the king with the royal crown, to

< 125 >

show off to the people." Queen Vashti refused and she was executed. Later, Achashverosh remembered his beautiful wife and became depressed.

In the Talmud *(Megillah 7b)* we read that Rava said: It is the duty of a man to mellow himself with wine on Purim until he cannot tell the difference between "cursed be Haman" and "blessed be Mordechai." Subsequently, Rava and R' Zeira joined together in a Purim feast. They indeed became mellow, and Rava arose and cut R' Zeira's throat.

Rabbeinu Ephraim, who is quoted by Rabbeinu Nissim, states that this narrative is presented in order to advise us that one should limit his intake of alcohol on Purim so that he does not reach such a level of intoxication. If these *gedolim* went amiss, how vigilant must common people be not to overindulge in alcohol.

On the other hand, the Torah never forbade alcohol. During the time of the Temple, there was daily *nisuch hayayin* (wine libations) with the sacrifices in the *Beis HaMikdash*. In fact, the Kiddush wine is an essential part of Shabbos and Yom Tov. It is fortuitous, too, to use wine for the *Havdalah* services to ensure long life. Moreover the Four Cups of Wine *(arba kosos)* are an integral part of the Pesach Seder, and wine is included in the proceedings under the *chuppah*, at *Sheva Brachos*, and at a *bris*.

Is a person immune to becoming drunk because he is drinking with the sincere intention of fulfilling a *mitzvah*? No way. There is no person who is immune to alcoholism. It is a disease, and we must go out of our way to protect ourselves from any disease.

< 126 >

Sam's Story

Sam was a well-respected member of the community and active in the *shul* where he *davened*. He was a hard-working accountant who put in long hours, especially during tax season, at the large firm where he was employed. The proud father of four children, Sam was dedicated to his family and a generous provider.

Sam did enjoy fine wines and a good vodka, but he never drank more than one or two shots at the *kiddush* in *shul* every Shabbos morning. When they attended a *simcha*, he was also mindful of his intake, since he was the driver and had no intention of giving over the wheel to anyone else on the way home.

Lately, though, some of his investments hadn't made out so well, which gave rise to financial concerns. By nature, Sam was a worrier and a stickler for perfection. He didn't like when the numbers didn't line up. He began to have trouble sleeping at night, and then he found it hard to get out of bed in the morning. Mornings were very tough, and he had to push himself to start the day and get to his desk at work

Sam kept hoping that things would get better and that his state of depression would diminish. But, as the weeks went by his melancholy escalated, and he was finding it more and more difficult to get through the day.

Although he had ordered food from a local restaurant to eat at his desk, Sam craved a snack when he arrived home. He headed into the kitchen to forage in the refrigerator. As he walked in, he espied a bottle of his favorite fine single-malt whiskey standing on the counter next to a freshly baked cake.

"That looks good," he thought to himself. "I'll pour myself a drink to take the edge off."

< 127 >

As the amber liquid made its way down his throat, Sam felt the warmth of the drink begin to do its magic. He took another few drinks, and felt himself relax, as the tension eased and his mood mellowed.

With a spring in his step, he went upstairs to bed and slept like a baby.

Sam went to work the next morning, none the worse for wear after his previous night's indulgence. In fact, when he recalled his good spirits, he contemplated making it his regular practice.

That night when he came home, he did exactly that. He had a few drinks to relax and enjoyed a good night's sleep. Things got much better, and Sam believed he had found the elixir for his misery. His pain was eased, his concerns were alleviated; he felt good.

His nightly assignations with the bottle remained a secret, but Sam's work began to slide. Sam was waking up late and misremembering appointments. His reputation for accuracy began to falter as his concentration and attention to detail were affected, and he was submitting work that was not up to par. When he came up for his quarterly review, glaring errors were revealed, and Sam was immediately put on probation.

Sam's self-esteem plummeted and he was, understandably, in very low spirits. His usual few drinks no longer sufficed at night, and now he had to consume an entire bottle before he could even consider going up to his bed.

At work, Sam was moody and unreliable. After a number of poor judgement calls at client meetings, his employer dismissed him. Totally in denial, Sam would not acknowledge any drinking problem. He told his wife the firm was downsizing, and heartily assured her that he would have no problem

< 128 >

finding another job.

With no job to wake up to in the morning, Sam began to sleep in late. He wasn't pursuing any employment opportunities. His despondency deepened and he began to drink more heavily. His addiction to alcohol was no longer a secret at home, but Sam had not yet hit bottom.

That happened when his sister's oldest daughter got married. Sam and his family came to the hall early to take part in the pictures, and Sam headed straight for the bar. Before the festivities were underway, Sam had already partaken of quite a few glasses. When the *mesader kiddushin* (officiating rabbi) finally arrived, an hour later than scheduled, everyone began to look for Sam because he was in charge of the *kibbudim* (honors). He was nowhere to be found, and the wedding ceeremony took place without him. After the *chuppah* (wedding ceremony) a more thorough search was launched and Sam was found passed out, behind the kitchen area outside the building.

Sam had to be rushed to the hospital, and his comedown became public knowledge. It was humiliating to say the least, but Sam was finally forced to confront his problem head on and admit that he was abusing alcohol.

The next days, weeks and months were exceptionally trying. Sam had a serious problem with alcohol, and he and his wife were experiencing a particularly strained relationship because of it and the concomitant consequences.

Sam had to work very hard to overcome his deeply negative emotions of shame and fear in order to facilitate his recovery. He and his wife spent months in therapy and attended Al Anon (AA) meetings three times weekly. It was a long and difficult road, with many ups and downs.

< 129 >

Sam incorporated more spirituality into his life by joining some of the classes and *shiurim* that were offered in the *shul.*

It took close to two years before Sam became sponsor of a new AA member. He remains sober, but continues to attend AA meetings and to maintain his commitment to *shiurim* and Torah classes.

• • •

< 130 >

Rabbi Nachman of Breslov says: Drunkenness causes a person to fall from his high position, to accept bribes, and to deny the truth.

Alcohol abuse presents a danger to people – physically, mentally and spiritually. One has to be vigilant in his adherence to the Torah command *(Devarim 4:15)* "*V'nishmartem me'od l'nafshoseichem* – you should be careful to protect the physical welfare of your bodies."

- Liver function can be damaged. It takes a few days for the liver to recover and resume normal functioning after a round of drinking.

- Too little sugar in the body can cause coma and seizures.

- The heart can beat so irregularly that it can stop.

- The body loses temperature causing hypothermia. If a person passes out in the cold, he can die.

- Alcohol ages and damages the brain.

- Prolonged drinking can cause pancreatitis.

- One of the most common causes of death from alcohol, especially among teens, is by choking on their vomit. Having blacked out from the alcohol overdose, they unconsciously breathe in their vomit, depriving their brain of oxygen.

- People are taking risks with alcohol if they drink and drive, operate machinery, mix alcohol with over-the-counter or prescription drugs, or have a medical condition that is exacerbated by drinking.

- People are risking others' lives if they drink alcohol while caring for children.

< 131 >

Alcohol decreases a person's inhibitions. When people drink too much they may do or say things they don't mean. Alcohol changes a person's ability to think, speak, and see things as they really are. This impairment also impacts negatively on a person's vigilance to guard against sin. That is one of the reasons for the various halachos that we have with regard to wine and drinking.

The Talmud in *Eruvin (65a)* states: The sale or purchase made by an intoxicated person is valid. If he committed a transgression under the influence of alcohol, even if he is liable the punishment of death or lashes, he receives that punishment. The rule is that he is regarded as a sober man and may only be exempt from prayer.

The *Acharonim* (later authorities) dispute the level of intoxication that determines one's responsibility.

The drunkenness of Lot puts one in the category of a *shoteh*– one who is mentally deficient – and he is therefore exempt from all *mitzvos*.

Rav Bar Rav Huna maintains that one who drank shouldn't pray, but if he prayed his *tefillos* are considered acceptable. One who is intoxicated is not in a position to *daven*; if he does, his *tefillah* is an abomination.

Our sages assert that one who drank can speak in front of the king, but one who is intoxicated is not able to address the king.

The halacha (the Jewish law) is that although one may not pray if he is intoxicated, he must recite the *Birchas HaMazon* (Grace After Meals) if he ate bread.

There are many halachos that are discussed with regard to one's state of intoxication. For example, if one is inebriated at

< 132 >

the time of *kiddushin* is his/her marriage binding?

The Rambam *(Hilchos Ishus, 4:18)* states that even if the individual is exceedingly drunk, the *kiddushin* is valid. But if his state of drunkenness is comparable to Lot's drunkenness then his *kiddushin* is not valid. That is one of the reasons why the *chassan* and *kallah* fast on the day of their wedding *(Teshuvas Maharam Mintz)*.

In a similar vein, the Rambam notes *(Hilchos Chovel U'Mazik 1:21)* that a person who damages something or wounds somebody – whether he is asleep or awake, whether it is inadvertent or deliberate, whether or not he is drunk – is liable to pay the damage.

The *Mishnah Berurah (695:4)* notes that one should ensure he is never so intoxicated that he cannot do his *avodah* (service of Hashem) properly, i.e. prayers, blessings, etc. The Yam Shel Shlomo adds that even if his intoxication is at the level of Lot's he is still liable to pay for all the damage he has imposed.

One has to know his limits and how much alcohol he can tolerate. It is known that when an individual would come to the great Sephardic Gaon, Baba Sali, for a *bracha*, the Baba Sali would offer the person a drink of Arak (a highly alcoholic drink that is more than 100-proof).

Once, the person seeking a *bracha* protested, saying, "My doctor told me I'm not allowed to have it."

Baba Sali insisted he could. "Don't worry; you can drink it."

The man poured himself a drink, downed it, and then picked up the bottle to pour another one.

Baba Sali stopped him and said, "I only took responsibility for one."

< 133 >

The Badchan

A while ago I attended a wedding, where the *mechutanim* had brought in a *badchan* (a scholarly comedian) to entertain the wedding party and be *mesamei'ach chassan v'kallah* (make the bride and groom happy). The *badchan* for the evening was internationally well known and at 1:00 AM everyone quickly found a seat – men on one side, women on the other – so that they could enjoy the performance.

It was easy to see how the *badchan* had earned such an outstanding reputation. It didn't take long before the entire gathering was doubled up with laughter. It was good-natured ribbing, and the *badchan* had a knack for making the most mundane incidents seem very funny.

In one of the skits the *badchan* presented he portrayed a *shikkur,* the classic drunk. The sketch was hilarious and the crowd roared with laughter.

However, I became aware that the individual sitting next to me was not laughing at all. In fact, he seemed ill-at-ease and was not in any way enjoying the sketch. As I turned my head, he said to me, "I only wish I could find this funny." Then, to my utter consternation, I saw tears roll down his face.

Indeed, for many people drunkenness is not funny. It's a very serious matter, because they face the challenge of remaining sober on a daily basis. We don't joke about unfortunate people who are not well. Perhaps we have to reevaluate our criteria, for drunkenness is not a laughing matter.

• • •

< 134 >

- A staggering half-a-million children in the United States ages 9-12 are addicted to alcohol.

- More than 3 million teenagers in the United States between the ages of 14-17 are problem drinkers.

- According to recent research, 62% of U.S. high school seniors reported that they have been drunk recently.

- In the United States, more than 2 million people per year drive "under the influence".

- About 18 million adults are addicted to alcohol.

- Only three to five percent of alcoholics are what we consider "bums." Most alcoholics are people like you and me. Anyone can become an alcoholic – young, old, rich, poor, single, married, employed, or out-of-work.

In the sixth *bracha* of the *Sheva Brachos*, we say, "Blessed are You, Hashem … who created joy and gladness … let there soon be heard in the cities of Yehuda and the streets of Yerushalayim the sound of joy and the sound of gladness, the voice of the groom and the voice of the bride, the sound of the grooms' jubilance from their canopies and of youths from their song-filled feasts."

The Avudraham cites *Yirmiyah (33:11)* as the source for this blessing, and focuses on the expression of *"une'arim mimishteh neginasam* – youths from their song-filled feasts [i.e. with wine]" that is recited. Since it is the *chassan*'s peers who are celebrating the wedding festivities, asks the Avudraham, wouldn't it be more correct to identify them as *"bachurim* – young men"?

The Avudraham notes that there is a concern that if the young men imbibe too freely they may become drunk, reckless and not conduct themselves properly. On the other hand, we are not concerned that children will behave inappropriately and sin.

< 135 >

Leon's Story

L eon was the oldest son in an upper middle class family who
had recently moved into a well-to-do area in the suburbs.
He was a new student in the ninth grade class of the Jewish
day school that all the children in that area attended. Although
Leon was a good student, he was socially inept and could not
make friends. In his desire to meet other people, he reached out
to many but his efforts were always rebuffed.

He was not included in any of the extracurricular activities,
and usually sat on the sidelines when his classmates played
sports. Leon spent Shabbos in his room reading, and during
vacation days he moped around the house.

Leon's parents were busy career people, and his younger
baby sister was cared for by a live-in nanny. Whenever his
parents were aware of his lack of friends, they would ask, "Why
aren't you out with the boys? Haven't you made any friends
yet?" Other than that, though, they didn't realize the extent of
his misery and desperation to make friends.

One day, when Leon arrived home from school and went
through the mail, he found an invitation addressed to him. It
was a Bar Mitzvah invitation from a classmate. He gave it a
cursory glance after opening and then went to discard it in the
garbage pail.

"Who sent you that invitation?" his mother called out.
"And why are you throwing it out?"

"It's just an invitation from a classmate. The rule is that
you have to invite everybody in the class to your *bar mitzvah*
celebration, even if you're not friends with him."

"So ...?" asked his mother.

< 136 >

"We're certainly not friends, and I don't enjoy sitting at the table with no one to talk to. I'm just not part of the group," Leon said softly.

Leon's mother kept encouraging him to go, assuring him that a social event – as opposed to the school setting – was a great opportunity to develop friendships. "I'm sure you'll find at least one person who will talk to you, and perhaps become a friend."

After much coaxing, Leon's mother convinced him to drop in for an hour at the *simcha* and then she would pick him up

Leon did not look forward to the evening. When he entered the luxurious hall, he quickly found his seating card, took note of the table number and proceeded to his allocated seat. Some older boys had been seated at his table, and they were enjoying drinks from the open bar.

He sat there wondering if anyone he knew from his own class would be seated at his table, when – to his utter surprise – one of the boys spoke up.

"Hey, you wanna join us? What could I get you from the bar?"

Leon had never partaken of **any** alcoholic drink and wasn't sure he would even like it. But this was the first time anyone had ever asked him to join their fun.

"Sure," he said, "Get me whatever you're having."

Leon sipped the drink. The initial taste was quite bitter, and the liquid burned as it made its way down his throat. He could not understand why anyone would want to drink this stuff. With the others at the table looking on, however, Leon grimaced slightly, and then swallowed the remainder of the

< 137 >

glass with one gulp.

"Looks like it's not your first time," one said gleefully, as the three boys watched the drink disappear down Leon's throat.

"Let's have some more."

Leon hadn't eaten since much earlier that day, so after one more drink he was feeling relaxed and sociable. After another two drinks, though, he felt a little nauseous and his vision was slightly blurred.

He excused himself from the table and headed down the hall for some fresh air. He was certainly glad to see his mother pull up, just as he opened the door to the street.

A little high, Leon reported that he had a great time. When they got home he told his mother that it had been a long day. He was tired, he said, and was going straight to bed.

Although he woke up with a hangover the next morning, he reveled in the memories of the companionship he had enjoyed.

A few weeks later, he ran across one of the boys who had been at the Bar Mitzvah celebration.

"Hey, Leon, why don't you come over to my house tomorrow night?"

Leon jumped at this unexpected prospect of having friends and went over the next night to join his new buddies.

He was surprised when all they did was sit around in the living room and drink beer. Leon imagined the beer was soda and found it a little more palatable. There were no parents home, and without any adult to supervise, the boys imbibed a seemingly endless amount. There certainly were a lot of empty

< 138 >

bottles lying around the floor when he left for home.

He barely made it through the front door when he vomited all over himself, the hallway floor, and the nearby furniture. His mother came running quickly, and Leon was terrified to tell her the truth. He groaned, "I must have caught a virus. I really feel sick."

Sympathetically, Leon's mother helped him up to his room and into his bed. He didn't have a temperature, but his pallor was ashen and he seemed quite weak. She went downstairs to clean up the mess and hoped he would be better in the morning.

A little groggy in the morning, Leon slept in, but by the next day he felt better and returned to school.

Once he had recuperated, Leon actually began to look forward to the evening get-togethers. He began to enjoy the jags and the opportunity to drown his loneliness and misery for a few hours.

The private drinking bouts remained a secret until the day when one of the teachers noticed the six bottles of beer in his locker. Leon's mother was immediately called down to the school.

"Unfortunately, when I confronted your son, he admitted that the bottles were his and he has been drinking," the principal asserted. "This is a serious problem and must be dealt with forthwith."

Leon's parents were disappointed. They had thought that Leon had finally made some friends and was beginning to develop a social life. Instead, he had met up with an unseemly clique of boys who had introduced him to drinking.

Baruch Hashem, Leon's problem was discovered before too

< 139 >

much damage had been done. Obviously, Leon needed intensive counseling to address the underlying causes of his problem. His parents also did their research to find an appopriate support group for teenagers to help him on the road to recovery.

• • •

< 140 >

Why Does an Adult Drink?

Growing up in a society/family/neighborhood where alcohol is everywhere is going to make it more likely for some people to develop alcoholism.

People who start drinking at an earlier age are more likely to develop a dependency on alcohol.

An alcoholic personality

- is unable to cope with frustration.
- is emotionally immature.
- has a competitive nature.
- is a perfectionist.
- has low self-esteem.
- has depressive tendencies.
- feels socially inferior.

An addict may want to experience a high because

- it takes him beyond his pain and makes him feel good.
- he feels he has power.
- it reduces stress and relaxes him.
- it lets him enter a fantasy world.
- it makes him feel more comfortable in social situations.

< 141 >

Why Do Kids Drink?

The most common reasons why kids begin to drink are:

- Peer pressure

- Bullying

- Rebellion

- Stress

- Low self-esteem

- Depression

- Anxiety

- Boredom

- Dysfunctional family life

< 142 >

Alcohol Is Taking Over Your Life ...

- if you have tried to stop drinking for a week but have not been successful.

- if you think about drinking all the time.

- if you feel guilty after drinking.

- if other people are commenting about your drinking.

- if you have to take a drink in the morning to get yourself going after drinking heavily the night before.

- if you hide your alcohol, or buy it at different stores so people will not know how much you are drinking.

- if you are having blackouts, or have no recall of what took place while you were drinking.

- if you are not fulfilling your responsibilities either at home or at work.

- if you are taking sick days because you have hangovers.

- if you are unusually passive or argumentative.

< 143 >

Help

The only way the addict can be helped is when he understands that only he/she can control his/her behavior.

The addict has to make a commitment to quit and take the necessary steps to achieve that goal.

The addict must join one of the treatment programs that are available in order to get the tools and support necessary to be able to quit.

JACS (Jewish Alcoholics, Chemically Dependent Persons and Significant Others) is a program of the Jewish Board of Family and Children's Services that offers a Jewish environment for Jewish alcoholics in their quest for recovery.

< 144 >

Spiritual Help

HaGaon HaRav Simcha Wasserman, the Rosh Yeshiva of Yeshivas Ohr Elchanan, wrote the following in reply to an individual who had recently been introduced to Torah and *mitzvos*:

"Now that you are beginning to follow the *mitzvos* you have to perform them slowly, one by one. You need guidance. The one principle I do know is that the first *mitzvah* – the most important one – is to be *kovei'a itim laTorah* – to establish set times to study Torah."

We learn that the *nazir* was accorded a status similar to a *kohen gadol* merely for abstaining from wine, not cutting his hair, and not attending funerals.

The Telshe Rosh Yeshiva, HaGaon HaRav Mordechai Gifter, questioned the ability of the *nazir* to achieve such a high spiritual level by simply accepting upon himself such minor abstentions.

Rav Gifter explained that these undertakings are not minor at all. Each act is a great exercise in self-control. The individual who can rein in his desires and govern his emotions is one who can aspire to be truly righteous.

Studies have indicated that being spiritual, or religious, may help people overcome their addictions. In fact, spirituality has been an important component of the alcohol recovery process for many years. It should be noted here that true spirituality is not simply keeping *mitzvos* by rote, but striving to strengthen one's awareness of Hashem and cultivating the optimal close relationship with Him. This embodies the Ramchal's opening statement in *Mesilas Yesharim*, "To enjoy His [Hashem's] proximity, His closeness, and to develop a true

< 145 >

relationship with Him."

In recent years, it has been reported in the *Journal of the American Academy of Child and Adolescent Psychiatry* that teens who have an active spiritual life are half as likely to become alcoholics as those who have no religious beliefs. The lead author of this report stated, "Alcoholism, in addition to being a biological disorder, is a spiritual disorder."

< 146 >

Gambling Addiction

< 147 >

Gambling Addiction

The Talmud (Berachos 43b) states, "One should not recline with a group of people who are unlearned. Why? Because he might be drawn after them."

David HaMelech begins the first chapter of Tehillim, "Praiseworthy is the man who has not walked in the counsel of the wicked, and has not stood in the path of the sinful, and has not sat in the session of scorners." The Aznayim L'Torah comments on the three different positions that man assumes here, i.e. walking, standing, and sitting. He notes that in the course of the day, man has many free hours that are not consumed with business and work – time that can be illspent in inappropriate company.

He may "walk in the counsel of the wicked" and be drawn into all sorts of criminal activities like robbery, thievery, and fraud.

Others may be discerning and not engage in criminal or illegal activity, per se, but they are not as vigilant about their adherence to the Torah laws. They "stand in the path of the sinful" and may transgress many of the Torah's mandates.

The third type of individual believes he is not doing anything wrong at all. He "sits in the session of scorners" and revels in the amusement, merriment and diversions of ne'er-do-wells and those who waste their days in idle pursuit.

Praiseworthy is one who does not join any of these three groups for, in truth, the Shechinah does not rest in their midst.

< 149 >

Eli's Story

Eli and Beth had only been married a little over a year, when Beth called my home late one summer evening. At first I could barely make out who was on the phone; all I could hear was soft sobbing. When I finally discerned that it was she, I tried to calm her down so that we could speak, but was unsuccessful. With great effort, she finally asked if we could meet to discuss her problem.

The next morning I greeted a downcast teary-eyed Beth, accompanied by an unenthusiastic, disgruntled Eli at her side. I was surprised to see two such unhappy individuals, as they had seemed to be a match made in heaven.

Beth had difficulty beginning her story, but by the time she finished her tale I was stunned.

She moaned painfully for a few moments then said, "Soon after we returned home from a week's stay at my cousin's house in California, we received a call asking if we happened to have seen my cousin's wallet that had contained quite a bit of cash and was now missing. I informed my relatives that I knew nothing about it. When I asked Eli, he too claimed to have no knowledge of it. Imparting that information, and thanking them once again for their hospitality a week earlier, I hung up and went about my business.

"Two weeks later, we were invited to dinner at my parents' home. The following morning, during my mother's routine call, she mentioned that she couldn't seem to find her diamond ring. When I inquired a few days later, she told me that she had searched the entire house but it was gone.

"I didn't think about these incidents any further or connect them in any way, until I went to the bank three weeks later to withdraw money from our savings account. When I tried

< 150 >

to withdraw $300, the teller informed me that there was only $50 currently in the account. I argued that was impossible and she must be mistaken because I knew there was over seven thousand dollars in that account. She then produced a printout which indicated that $7,200 had been withdrawn over the past two weeks."

I glanced at Eli, but he was neither making eye contact with me, nor looking at Beth. He was staring studiously at the floor as though it was a puzzle he was trying to solve.

Beth struggled to continue. "I ran home in tears and waited for Eli to come home. When he finally came in, I asked if he was aware that $7,200 had been withdrawn from the account. He turned red and began to stammer. He finally confessed that he had hoped I would not find out about it because he had needed the money for an urgent matter. He said he knew what he was doing and I should trust him. He then assured me that the money would be replaced shortly.

"As time went on, though, I noticed that bills were not being paid. Whenever I would bring this up, Eli would tell me that he was broke. At this point, Rabbi Goldwasser, I don't even think Eli goes to work regularly."

There was a long silent pause. Eli was totally disengaged, Beth was overwhelmed with grief, and I – realizing the gravity of the situation – considered how to proceed.

I finally looked up and asked, "Eli, what is Beth saying? Do you know what she is implying?"

Defensively, Eli responded, "So I like to gamble a little bit. I don't know what the fuss is about. It's nothing heavy. It's just to pass time, like going bowling."

As do all problem gamblers, Eli insisted on minimizing

< 151 >

the problem. We discussed his "pastime" for a while, until Eli was compelled to admit that it was much more than a leisure activity. Eli revealed that he had been gambling heavily for the past few months. In fact, he had missed too much time from his job because of it and had been fired. He confessed that he owed an enormous sum of money to the wrong people and, out of desperation, he had resorted to "lifting" a few valuables.

Eli reassured both Beth and me that everything would be fine. It was just a phase and he would quit immediately. Frankly, though, quitting problem gambling is not the difficult part. It's remaining in recovery that is the major struggle.

Indeed, as the weeks went on, Eli's gambling became more excessive. He would gamble at a casino until the wee hours of the morning and not return until the following day.

Beth dragged Eli once more to my office. Eli was apologetic but not contrite, and said, "Rabbi, you don't understand. I just do it as a thrill. You cannot imagine the adrenaline rush when the roulette wheel is spinning, the excitement when my number is drawing near, or the charge when the cards are shuffled to begin a new game of blackjack."

In Eli's mind he was just having fun. "I have been scoring some big winnings. I just know that soon I will win enough for us to retire and then I'll quit this for good."

"Uh, oh," I said to myself. It is a fact that the winning streaks only become a justification for increased gambling as the addict starts to enjoy the high that it is providing and is imbued with a strong urge to return and win more.

"Eli," I said, "let's get real. You have a **major** problem." I pointed to all the things that had gone wrong. I quoted the statistics that the average debt incurred by a male pathological gambler in the United States is between $55,000 and $90,000;

< 152 >

the average rate of divorce for compulsive gamblers is nearly double that of non-gamblers; and 65% of gamblers commit crimes to support their gambling habit.

Although Eli seemed to be reconsidering the situation, he emphatically stated, "I'm not going to any gambler's therapy group, so you can forget about that!"

I felt that we had exhausted Eli's capacity to listen to much more that day, so we scheduled another session.

Emotions flew high as I tried to get Eli to understand the severity of his problem and the havoc it was already wreaking in his life. It took quite a while but after many sessions I finally got Eli to agree to do two things: First, he would attend one meeting of Gamblers Anonymous, and second, he would undertake a program of strengthening his connection to Hashem, through learning and *davening*.

If you're wondering how I was able to convince Eli to go to the Gamblers Anonymous meeting, that was very simple. I bet him two to one that he wouldn't go!

• • •

< 153 >

Compulsive or addicted gamblers are powerless to control their impulse to gamble. They keep gambling despite the hurt and pain they are causing their family and themselves. Gambling affects more than 15 million people.

Pathological gamblers are not exclusively male; the addiction crosses gender lines. The only difference lies in the type of gambling activities they join. Men tend to enjoy the excitement of casino gambling, e.g. blackjack or poker, whereas women engage in less interpersonal betting such as bingo, slot machines or internet activities. Research also indicates that unlike women, men tend to develop this disorder during their early teenage years. However, when women become addicted to gambling, the disorder escalates at a much faster pace than in men.

In addition to risking ruined marriages, lost careers, financial problems, bankruptcy, and trouble with the law, there are many *issurim* (Torah prohibitions) that one transgresses when engaging in gambling.

The activity of gambling itself is considered to be in the realm of *geneivah* – stealing.

The Mishnah *(Sanhedrin 24b)* cites categories of people who are unfit to bear witness and includes dice players and pigeon flyers, i.e. gamblers. R' Yehuda states gamblers are ineligible to testify when gambling is their only business; otherwise, they may be eligible. Rashi explains that R' Yehuda's opinion is that gamblers are not involved in doing anything useful and have no knowledge of basic business law, whereas one who has another occupation is sufficiently knowledgeable in this area.

The Talmud then cites a dispute between R' Bar Chama and R' Sheishes.

R' Bar Chama is of the opinion that gambling is an

< 154 >

asmachta of stealing – each player consents to the terms of the game because he expects to win. Consequently, when the loser must surrender his money to the winner it is not done wholeheartedly, and the winner is effectively considered to be stealing the winnings. He is therefore ineligible to be a witness or a judge.

R' Sheishes is of the opinion that gambling is not considered an *asmachta* of stealing because the players know that the winner is determined solely by chance and personal skill has no bearing on the outcome of the game. Therefore, he is surrendering his loss willingly. Nevertheless, he maintains that a gambler is not eligible to testify because he is not a productive member of society.

The Rambam *(Hilchos Gezeilah V'aveidah 6:10)* classifies gambling as robbery because he didn't do anything in order to acquire the money, i.e. he obtained the money from his friend without earning it, and in a frivolous manner.

Often the gambler depends on others for money to resolve dire financial situations that result because of losses incurred with gambling. If he is unsuccessful in bankrolling his activities by borrowing or begging, the gambler actually must resort to criminal acts (for example, stealing, fraud or forgery) in order to finance his gambling activities.

As was mentioned above, gambling is an unproductive pursuit, which is counter to our mandate to be industrious and fruitful *(Iyov 5:7)*, "For man is born to toil." Our sages tell us *(Sanhedrin 99b)* that the intent is that one was created to labor in Torah. A Jew is meant to spend his free time involved in meaningful activities such as Torah studies and the performance of *mitzvos* and *ma'asim tovim* (good deeds). To squander valuable time in vacuous pursuits instead of engaging in Torah study is indeed unwise.

< 155 >

There is a *mitzvas aseh* (positive command) in the Torah to learn Torah. The Rambam *(Hilchos Talmud Torah 3:3)* states that there is no *mitzvah* that is equal to that of Torah study. "Rather, Torah study is equal to all of the *mitzvos* together, for study leads to practice."

R' Tarfon states in *Ethics of Our Fathers (2:20)*, "The day is short; the task is abundant ..." The Medrash Shmuel comments that a person should not calculate the time he has to accrue his accomplishments in terms of a 120-year life span. Rather, he should constantly evaluate: What am I doing today?

The Navi Yeshayah cries out *(5:18)*, "Woe to those who pull misdeeds upon themselves with cords of falsehood, and sin like the ropes of a wagon."

R' Assi explains *(Sanhedrin 99b)* that initially temptation presents like a spider's thread, but eventually it is heavy like the ropes of a wagon. Rashi elaborates that at the outset it is possible that a person may be able to resist the temptation to sin because the cords are still thin, i.e. they are easily broken. However, as time goes on, and the individual concedes to temptation, he finds that he is bound to the sin with heavy cords that are much more difficult to sever.

HaGaon HaRav Aharon Kotler observes that misdeeds and sin develop and progress from that first misstep that one makes. An individual thinks to himself, "What harm can this minor infraction cause? What will I forfeit if I fritter away some time?"

The Vilna Gaon once saw a group of indolent people sitting around a table playing cards, engaged in idle chatter and bantering. As troubled as the Gaon was by their gambling activity, he was more concerned about their accountability in the Heavenly Court after 120 years. He noted that in the future when they are judged by the Heavenly Tribunal they would

< 156 >

undoubtedly be questioned about their gambling pastime. More importantly, though, he observed, they would be held liable for all the many hours that they idled away and didn't learn Torah.

The pathological gambler:

- Wants to have wealth and material goods without working hard to get them
- Thinks that money is both the cause of and solution to all of his problems
- Is often generous to the point of extravagance
- Is confident that he can beat the system and continues betting until he has lost all his money

HaGaon HaRav Aryeh Levine, who merited seeing many miracles performed for him, was asked why he never bought lottery tickets. He gave a surprising answer: "I'm afraid I might win." A person with a truly enlightened perspective doesn't even desire unearned riches, especially if he recalls the words of our sages (*Avos 2:7*), "The more possessions the more worry."

The Torah commands us (*Vayikra 19:2*), "Kedoshim tiheyu – you shall be holy." The Ramban explains this to mean "sanctify yourself by withdrawing from that which is permissible to you." This directive implies going beyond the strict observance of halachic law to encompass a broader adherence to halachic values. Thus, the gambler who is ensconced in the casino, surrounded by promiscuity and immodesty would, in essence, be sidestepping the issue of *kedoshim tiheyu*.

In the first chapter in *Tehillim*, David HaMelech writes, "Praiseworthy is the man who has not walked in the counsel of the wicked, and has not stood in the path of the sinful, and has not sat in the session of scorners. His desire is in the Torah of Hashem, and he meditates in His Torah day and night." The Minchas Yitzchak includes those who play dice and other games in the category of "scoffers."

< 157 >

Seth's Story

Seth was a fun-loving, adventurous guy who had always been a risk-taker, even when he was young. Teachers and counselors were always a little nervous when Seth was around because he never hesitated to take someone up on a dare. When one of the older students challenged Seth to climb up the school flagpole, he shimmied up to the top and back down before the principal ever made out it of the school building. When he got his hot new sports car, he joined some guys in drag racing, until that pastime petered out.

During his high school years in yeshiva, Seth was not a serious learner. He was an average student, but his high spirits and dauntlessness made him one of the most popular guys in school.

When he left school, Seth became a salesman. He was actually quite successful and had recently earned the company's "Salesman of the Year" award. A few weeks earlier a *shadchan* had set him up with a young lady and their relationship had been developing nicely. Seth was hopeful that they would be an engaged couple soon. Seth's evenings were his own, though. Once in a while he would attend a Torah lecture, but his activities were generally of a more recreational nature. He developed a particular affinity for poker, and worked to improve his game.

One of his friends had introduced him to "the club" – a group of guys who met regularly in a basement in Brooklyn for pizza, drinks, and a good game of poker. They were an eclectic group but definitely an interesting one. He noticed that some of the players took their game very seriously; this was no mere pastime for them. The game would begin at 10:00 in the evening, but usually not end till 3:30 in the morning. They would then sit around in the local coffee shop till the wee hours of the morning.

< 158 >

The privacy of the group, the passion of the game, the dynamics of the players, and the amount of money at stake were all intriguing, and Seth looked forward each time to the next evening they would meet.

The schedule was very tiring for someone like Seth, who worked during the day. But he could not resist the temptation to bet and to play the odds. Because of the inherent nature of his job and the irregular hours it entailed, though, Seth was able to keep his job, because he was still an innate natural at sales.

Motzoei Shabbos, especially, was a very busy night when there were two games playing simultaneously – one consisting of professionals and the other for the rookies. It was a guaranteed all-nighter and a nail-biter for those with much money to lose.

Seth's life, as he had known it, began to crumble around the edges. It was difficult to function on only a few hours of sleep, so Seth stayed in bed a little longer each morning and missed *davening shacharis* with a *minyan*. When he did get out of bed, he barely had the time to put on his *tefillin;* sometimes he just neglected the rite. If he was running late at work, he would from time to time skip *maariv* at night as well. His *tefillah* became a hit-or-miss option.

The young lady he had been seeing also noticed a change in Seth. He would nod off in middle of a conversation, and often could not recall what they had discussed on their previous date. He seemed preoccupied at times and offered lame apologies for his inattentiveness. He always had a cup of coffee in his hand, and popped the No-Doz tablets like candy. Seth did not seem to be the steady, reliable young man and partner in life that she had been seeking.

Despite the fact that his future was on the line, Seth could not disassociate from the night life he had discovered. He was an accepted member of "the club." The thrill and excitement of

< 159 >

the game was seductive and addictive.

It was Sunday at midnight, about one hour into the game. Suddenly, a loud voice on a bullhorn intruded and broke the silence of the night. "You are completely surrounded. Come out with your hands raised above your head!"

Seth looked around at the others, and noticed that many did not seem fazed. He, however, was horror-struck. He was a young man, with no police record. Although there may have been a subconscious awareness that "the club" was operating illegally, Seth was not prepared to be part of a dramatic arrest. He put his head down on the table and began to cry.

"Hey, Seth, you better haul your body out there, or they're going to come in and drag you out!" one of his partners-in-crime called out.

Seth emerged from the basement and was blinded by the floodlights that lit up the entire area like it was day. There were news reporters with their cameras rolling, microphones in their hands, reporting the breakup of the gambling ring. Apparently, some of the "interesting" players in the game had already been arrested before on illegal gambling charges and were now in violation of their parole agreement.

Seth was in serious trouble. He was fingerprinted, had his photo taken and was put into a cell until he could get a lawyer and post bail. Seth's picture was in all the newspapers, his *yarmulke* in plain view. One paper ran a headline: "Orthodox Gambler Offers Prayers to Win."

The young woman Seth had been dating felt betrayed and hurt beyond words. How could she have spent all those evenings with such a loser and not seen through him?

As Seth sat in his cell overnight, he cried even more. It

< 160 >

wasn't only his extreme humiliation that pained him. His anguish was intensified because of an oath he had made many years earlier when his father had abandoned the family. Seth had sworn that he would never walk in his father's shoes. His father had been a lifelong gambler who had clashed with the law one too many times.

• • •

< 161 >

Gambling is a major source of marital conflict. The effects of pathological gambling are often devastating for spouses and children, as family is neglected and financial problems mount. Studies also indicate a high rate of physical and/or emotional abuse among problem gamblers.

Shalom is an essential theme in Torah life. *Shalom* is one of the names of Hashem, the name of the Jewish nation, and the name of Mashiach *(Derech Eretz Zuta, Perek HaShalom)*.

The Medrash *(Bamidbar Rabbah 11:18)* relates, "Great is the peace that is bestowed upon those who learn Torah ... great is the peace that Hashem's name is Peace." The Zohar *(1:90)* comments that when Hashem commands the *Kohanim* to bless the Jewish nation He says, *(Bamidbar 6:23)*, "*Koh sevarchu* – so you shall bless." The word *koh* is numerically equivalent to twenty-five alluding to the twenty-five times that the word "peace" is mentioned in the Torah. So great is the blessing of peace, including *shalom bayis* (domestic harmony).

In fact, our sages note that there are times when certain laws are revoked in order to ensure that harmony is maintained between husband and wife. For example, the Torah states that when Sarah learned that she and Avraham would have a son, Sarah laughed at the notion, reflecting that she and Avraham were already old *(Bereishis 18:12)*. Yet when Hashem spoke to Avraham, He only relayed Sarah's reaction concerning herself. Bar Kaparah states: How great is peace that the Torah altered her words *(Yalkut Shimoni)*. The Talmud notes that, in the *parsha* of an *isha sotah*, the Torah permits the holy name of Hashem to be erased in the water in order to reinstate harmony between husband and wife *(Chulin 141a)*.

There is a *mitzvas lo sa'aseh* (prohibition) of *bal tashchis* (lit. do not destroy) which, the Rambam explains *(Hilchos Melachim 6:10)*, includes senseless damage, misuse or waste. This precept has its roots in the Torah command not to destroy fruit-bearing trees when besieging a city in war *(Devarim 20:19)*.

< 162 >

The compulsive gambler is initially seduced by that first big win, and keeps returning to cash in on his "golden touch." However the odds of winning when gambling are exceedingly slim, and eventually the addict's goal is to at least recoup his losses. At this point the compulsive gambler is literally throwing good money after bad – suffering irretrievable losses and accumulating huge debts.

One may wonder if a gambler should make a vow to stop gambling.

In general, Jewish law discourages one from making a *neder,* a vow. In the Talmud *(Taanis 11a)* R' Elazar HaKappar questions why the *pasuk (Bamidbar 6:11)* states that the *nazir* must bring a *korban* to "provide him atonement for having sinned...." What was his sin? His answer is that it refers to the fact that he denied himself wine. The inference is made that if a person who only deprived himself of wine is called a sinner, how much more is one who denies himself the enjoyment of other permissible pleasures.

One of the situations in which it is permitted to make a vow is if a person is fearful of transgressing a *mitzvah (Yoreh Dei'ah 203:7).*

The Rashba cites the question of a gambler who made a *neder* that he would abstain from gambling for a specified amount of time. However, he found it virtually impossible to abide by his oath and wanted to be absolved from his *neder.*

The Rashba answered that he could not be released from his oath. First of all, gambling is already prohibited by the Torah, and we could not grant the individual permission to transgress. Secondly, we would not want to transgress one prohibition so that the individual does not transgress a different prohibition.

The *Shulchan Aruch (Yoreh Dei'ah 228:15)* quotes the following:

< 163 >

"We do not annul a vow that was made to prohibit a forbidden activity. Even a vow that forbids an activity that is only rabbinically prohibited should not be annulled. For instance, a vow not to gamble should not be annulled."

In his *Sefer Machane Yisrael*, the Chofetz Chaim vehemently disapproves of gambling activities and points out a few of the Torah transgressions one will breach.

There is the sin *(aveirah)* of speaking *devarim beteilim* – idle chatter. When a person is sitting in the casino, or playing cards, he is not usually conversing about business or important matters. The players are generally laughing, bantering and joking. The Chofetz Chaim cites the Talmud *(Yuma 19b)*, "Rava said: One who engages in idle chatter transgresses a positive command."

There is an *aveirah* of speaking *nivul peh* – profanity. Inevitably, the longer the players sit around, the repartee is reduced to vulgarity and bad language. The Chofetz Chaim cites various sources in the Talmud that denounce this conduct. We learn in *Avodah Zarah (18b)*, "He who scoffs, affliction will befall him … his sustenance will be reduced …. he will fall into *gehennom*…brings destruction upon the world." In *Shabbos (33a)*, we are cautioned, "As a punishment for obscenity, troubles multiply, cruel decrees are newly proclaimed, the youth of Israel die, the fatherless and widows cry out and are not answered … even if a sentence of seventy years' happiness has been sealed for him, it is reversed for evil … *gehennom* is made deeper for him." Our sages further caution us that even the one who listens to this perverse speech and remains silent will suffer the same fate.

There is the strong concern about *"asmachta"* (discussed earlier). This often precipitates heavy drinking and brawling among the players, which tends to lead to the transgression of many other Torah and rabbinic prohibitions.

< 164 >

Aaron's Story

Aaron was your average yeshiva-cum-working man, all-around kind of guy. He had a well-paying job in the city, kept a learning *seder* every night, and played ball with his buddies on Sunday morning. He and his wife, Chana, had been married for three years and had a little girl. Chana worked at a service agency that was closer to home and was usually home by 5:00 PM. Their life had settled into a routine of domestic bliss and everything seemed to be going well.

It was Friday afternoon on a bitterly cold day in December as Chana hurriedly rushed around the kitchen to finish her preparations for Shabbos. Aaron had spent the night out-of-town after a two-day meeting with clients in Boston that had lasted late into the night, and Chana had expected him home no later than 1:00 in the afternoon. Now, as she glanced up at the clock, she realized that she had not heard from Aaron in a few hours and it was barely a half hour to Shabbos. When she called his cell, it went directly to voice mail. She was surprised and slightly concerned because Aaron never turned his phone off when he was in the car. Her unease escalated to alarm as the minutes ticked by on the clock and it was five minutes to candle-lighting time.

Just as she went into the dining room to light the candles, the phone rang. Chana quickly ran to the phone, fearing the worst. Aaron was on the phone and he sounded upset.

"Chanie, I don't know what happened! As I was driving I felt myself nodding off. I was just so exhausted that I pulled off the road for a fifteen-minute nap and it seems I slept for more than two hours. When I woke up and started driving I must have made a wrong turn somewhere, but I got hopelessly lost. I knew I would not be able to make it home for Shabbos." Aaron sounded quite upset.

< 165 >

"Where will you stay? What will you eat?" Chana worriedly asked.

"Don't worry," Aaron reassured her. "When I saw how late the hour was I quickly drove up to a supermarket and bought some stuff. Then I pulled into a motel off the highway and checked in. I'll be fine, but I will miss you and the baby."

Shabbos night Aaron came home quite late. Chana wanted to ask him some questions, but Aaron claimed he was totally wiped and just flopped into bed and went to sleep. Chana was curious about how Aaron had spent a lonely Shabbos in the middle of nowhere, but Aaron seemed less than anxious to discuss it, and was on the run – *davening* and *seder*, the ball game with the guys. By the end of the day, life had moved on.

Everything remained on an even keel, until one day a non-Jewish associate of Chana, who worked out of a different office, stopped by Chana's desk.

"How're you doing, Chana? I didn't know your husband is a player!"

"A player for what?" asked Chana innocently.

"A player, like playing the odds – you know. I saw your husband in Atlantic City the last time I was there. It was a Friday afternoon and your husband was at the blackjack table."

"You've got to be kidding me," Chana joked with her. "My husband is not a gambler. He would never hang out in a casino."

"Hey, just calling it like I see it!" exclaimed the co-worker. "I recognized him from the picture you keep on your desk. I'm great at faces, and I'm sure it was him."

< 166 >

Although Chana kept on insisting that it was a case of mistaken identity, she couldn't shake the thought that there was a possibility that her co-worker was telling the truth. To be honest, Chana could not deny the fact that she had never really heard the whole story from Aaron about that fateful Friday.

Chana, being the good wife that she was, did not want to rock the boat, so she quickly buried the conversation in the recesses of her mind and tried very hard to forget all about it.

A few weeks later, as Chana went through the pockets of some clothing she was taking to the cleaners, she came across a receipt from that casino her co-worker had visited in Atlantic City. Dismayed, her mouth went dry as she collapsed on the bed. Could her co-worker have, indeed, been correct? Had she truly seen Chana's husband in the casino that Friday afternoon? Was it actually possible that Aaron had lied to her about where he had spent Shabbos?

As all these thoughts ran through her head, Chana realized that it was very possible that she did not know her husband at all, and she was married to a complete stranger.

Chana was in a fog for the next few hours, as she fed their little girl supper, played with her for a while, bathed her and then put her to bed. Then Chana sat down at the dining room table, and patiently waited for her husband to return home from work.

"Aaron, we must talk," Chana said calmly as soon as Aaron came through the door. Aaron was a little taken aback, but he put his briefcase down on the floor, hung up his coat in the closet, and then sat down at the other end of the dining room table.

"Aaron," began Chana, "that Friday afternoon when you called that you were too far from home, did you happen to

< 167 >

ultimately spend Shabbos in an Atlantic City hotel?"

At first Aaron vehemently denied any knowledge of what she was talking about. Chana resolutely kept questioning him until Aaron broke down. "I was going to tell you. I really was going to tell you. I didn't want to lie to you," he cried. Chana wasn't sure what was more upsetting – seeing a grown man sobbing bitterly in defeat or knowing that her husband had lied to her about something so important.

Aaron tried to explain. "One of my colleagues who had accompanied me to Boston cajoled me to join him for a few throws of the dice. As you know, it's been very busy at the office and I've been under a lot of pressure lately, driven by the clients and management. I figured it would be a good way to let off some steam and relax a bit. Of course, I only planned to spend an hour or two, but then I lost some money and I desperately wanted to recover it. So I kept trying my hand again and again at the roulette table; I just couldn't control myself. I felt powerless in my drive to recoup my losses.

"Honestly, Chanie, I felt terrible about skipping out on you like that for Shabbos. But I promise it was a freak occurrence. I've been feeling terrible about it, and it won't happen again."

Aaron's credibility had been destroyed, but Chana desperately wanted to believe him. It was difficult for her to conceive that Aaron was not the man she married, so Chana accepted his apology. Aaron also promised to work very hard to regain Chana's trust.

However, a few weeks later when Chana reviewed the monthly bank statement she noticed a number of evening cash withdrawals had been made. Shortly after their marriage, Chana and Aaron had set up a budget plan and as far as Chana knew there were no extra funds available for casual spending. When Chana questioned Aaron about these withdrawals he

< 168 >

explained that he had borrowed some cash during the day and he promised to go to an ATM machine to pay it back on the way home from work.

That was about the time the minor peculiarities and incongruities that Chana encountered every once in a while began to frighten her. Chana noticed that Aaron would often not buy all the groceries itemized on her list. When she would send him shopping for Shabbos he would scrimp, and only buy one or two treats she had requested.

One day when she got into the car, she found fifty lottery tickets stuffed under the seat. Chana stared in horror at the worthless pieces of paper, as she thought of the food that they supposedly couldn't afford to buy.

Chana could no longer deny the evidence in front of her. Aaron was a compulsive gambler and he was unwilling to admit it to himself and to her.

This time when Chana spoke to Aaron she was very firm. There would be no discussion of compromises or negotiation. She presented a comprehensive plan of action to address his problem head-on. They immediately set up an appointment with a therapist who recommended joining Gamblers Anonymous and Gam-Anon for Aaron and Chana respectively. Chana attended the meetings regularly, as did Aaron ostensibly.

Although Aaron was definitely contrite, Chana suspected that Aaron had not completely turned his back on his gambling activities. There were times during the day when he was incommunicado. There were days he would come home very late in the evening complaining about his heavy workload. Nor was Chana certain that Aaron was truly ready to admit that his compulsion to gamble had the better of him.

< 169 >

In fact, Aaron's activities had become a threat to the wellbeing of his family. One afternoon when Chana returned from work the front door of their apartment was unlocked. Thinking that her husband had come home early and forgotten to lock the door behind him, she walked in. To her shock and dismay, two complete strangers were comfortably seated on the living room couch, as if they owned the place.

One of the men slowly rose out of his chair and, with a menacing finger pointed at Chana, said, "Mrs. C., your husband owes us a few thousand dollars. We suggest that he pay that back promptly." Without further ado, the two men walked slowly out the door, leaving a traumatized and stunned Chana behind.

Chana hurriedly ran out of the house and picked up her daughter at the babysitter. As she drove to her parents' home she called Aaron and left a message on his phone that she would not be returning because his gambling activities were now endangering the family's safety.

Aaron began to understand the severity of his situation and realized he had hit rock bottom. He grasped the reality that there was a very good possibility that he would lose his family forever if he did not clean up his act.

Aaron immediately set aside any feelings of shame he had and called his Rav. With the help of knowledgeable professionals, he was directed to a therapist who could work with him one-on-one. He also joined a support group for compulsive gamblers. Some basic ground rules were developed to help Aaron maintain his commitment to stay away from gambling. A system was established whereby Aaron was accountable for every hour of the day and had to check in regularly with certain people to report on his activities.

By making an independent conscious decision to quit,

< 170 >

Aaron had finally taken that crucial first step in overcoming his gambling addiction. Although there is a lot of work still to be done, Aaron is well aware of what is at stake.

• • •

< 171 >

Red Flags

The compulsive gambler often exhibits specific characteristics that may be red flags indicating a serious problem.

- He escapes into the fantasy world of gambling because he is unable or unwilling to accept reality.

- He has an unrealistic desire to attain the good things in life without working for them.

- He fantasizes about his "big win" and the luxurious gifts he will be able to bestow on families and friends.

- He needs to feel "in control."

Are You Addicted?

- You feel most secure at the gambling table despite an inner awareness that you are destroying your life.

- You are secretive or defensive about your gambling.

- You are increasingly desperate to find money to fund the gambling, and have even resorted to stealing jewelry or other items that can be easily pawned.

- You gamble until you have spent your last dollar.

- You repeatedly try to stop or cut back on your gambling activities.

- The thrill of the game overshadows all other considerations.

< 172 >

Help

As with any addiction, successful treatment programs for pathological gamblers work one day at a time. It is important to incorporate cognitive and behavioral modification therapy with a support group, such as Gamblers Anonymous. It is also recommended that gamblers, and their family, receive credit counseling and/or assistance with money management issues.

To succeed in his recovery, the compulsive gambler must learn to be able to identify the triggers that activate the gambling urge. He must then work on eliminating them from his life and/or finding alternative behaviors to keep him from gambling. The compulsive gambler must also make certain to remove himself from situations that facilitate or impel his habit.

Overcoming a gambling addiction is a difficult process. Although the ultimate decision to quit belongs to the gambler, it is critical for the problem gambler to have the support of family and friends.

Individuals who find that gambling provides the rush of adrenaline they desire, need to engage in a sport, a challenging hobby, or an exerting session of exercise that will impart a similar pleasure.

If boredom, loneliness or too much time on one's hands takes him to the nearest casino, the recovering addict must schedule recreational time with family or friends, find other enjoyable pastimes and diversions, or join a social group that shares his interests.

The inveterate gambler must completely divest himself from all control of family finances. He should only have access to a limited amount of cash at all times and not own any credit cards.

Gaming establishments, when notified, are often helpful by limiting the gambler's betting at their casinos.

< 173 >

Spiritual Help

As in all other areas of life, the Torah delineates what is permissible and what is forbidden in the areas of financial transactions, business activities, the acquisition of money and its disbursement.

The Talmud *(Kesubos 67b)* relates that a poor man once came to Rava for *tzedakah*.

Rava asked him, "What do your meals consist of?"

The beggar replied, "I eat a fattened hen and aged wine."

Rava questioned, "Did you not consider the burden that places on the community to provide for you?"

"Do I eat from theirs?" the man asked. "I eat from the food of Hashem, as it says [*Tehillim 145:15*], 'The eyes of all look to You with hope, and You give them their food in its proper time.' It is noted that the *pasuk* states, 'in its time' and not 'in their time,' indicating that each and every person is allotted his sustenance from Hashem in accordance with his needs and his preferences."

As they were speaking, Rava's sister – whom he had not seen in thirteen years – arrived with a fattened hen and aged wine.

"How remarkable!" exclaimed Rava. He then turned to the beggar and said, "I apologize to you; I spoke too much. Come and eat."

We learn that a person must strengthen his *emunah* in Hashem, for He will provide the individual with all his needs, as it says further in *Tehillim*, "You open Your hand, and satisfy the desire of every living thing." The knowledge and unwavering faith that everything is from Hashem obviates any need to

< 174 >

indulge in get-rich-quick schemes such as gambling.

The Torah also teaches us that possessions and wealth are not just meant as an accumulation of material belongings. We are directed to allocate money for charitable purposes, to sustain the poor, to support the study and dissemination of Torah, and to give *ma'aser*. The Torah encourages us to use our wealth for altruistic and humanitarian causes instead of engaging in selfish expenditures. Charity has the power to elevate the soul and increases G-d's blessing for wealth, as the Talmud tells us *(Shabbos 119a)*, "Give charity so that you may prosper."

If one is experiencing financial difficulty or wants to become wealthy, his salvation will not be found in the casinos or at the race track. Hashem is our source of wealth, as it says *(Chaggai 2:8)*, "Mine is the silver and mine is the gold, the word of Hashem." Our duty is to follow all the Torah's mandates with regard to money. The *Shulchan Aruch Choshen Mishpat*, written by R' Yosef Karo (1488-1575), specifically addresses in great detail issues of ethical business conduct and honesty in financial transactions.

Shlomo HaMelech writes in *Koheles (4:6)*, "Better is one handful of pleasantness than two fistfuls of labor and striving after wind." The *Medrash Rabbah* explains: "Superior is the one who gives a small amount of charity from his own possessions than one who robs or obtains his money dishonestly or illegally and then gives large amounts of charity from that which actually belongs to others. "Striving after wind" alludes to one who seeks approbation and homage (for his philanthropy).

The Hebrew word for money is *mamon* and its numerical value is equivalent to the Hebrew word for ladder, *sulam*. Money is simply a tool that can be used for good or bad. Utilizing his money appropriately, as a Torah Jew, man can rise to the highest heights; conversely, if he uses his money imprudently or unwisely, counter to the Torah's directives, he can spiritually hit rock-bottom.

< 175 >

Shopping Addiction

< 177 >

Shopping Addiction

The Talmud relates (Tamid 32b) a fascinating story about Alexander of Macedon who, along his travels, sat by a well and began to eat. He had with him some salted fish that he washed off with the well water, and when he did so they released a sweet odor. Alexander of Macedon observed that this indicated that the well came from Gan Eden. He walked alongside the water until he came to the door of Gan Eden.

When he wanted to enter, he was told that only the righteous could enter. He replied, "I too am a king; I am also of some account," and he requested a memento. They gave him an eyeball.

He then proceeded to weigh all his gold and silver against the eyeball, and the eyeball weighed less.

He asked the sages, "How could this be?"

They replied, "It is the eyeball of a human being, which is never satisfied with all the riches."

Rashi notes that this alluded to Alexander himself who despite the vast wealth and land he had amassed constantly sought more lands to conquer and more possessions to acquire.

Alexander of Macedon asked, "How can you prove that this is so?"

The sages took a little dust and covered the eyeball, and immediately it was weighed down. That is as it says (Mishlei 27:20), "As the grave and gehennom are not satiated, so the eyes of man are never satiated."

< 179 >

Dina's Story

Dina loved shopping. Since the time she was a little girl she had loved going into the stores, picking out dresses and shoes, bringing home her purchases, and wearing her new apparel. She never got tired of it!

As a matter of fact, as she entered her teenage years, she found herself spending many hours of the day at the mall, making numerous purchases, and coming home with bags and bags of stuff that she had purchased. She always seemed to need something new! No matter how many clothes there were in her closet and in her drawers, no matter how many shoes were neatly arranged in the shoe bag, (and then on the shelves, and under her bed, in their shoeboxes), she always found another outfit and another pair of shoes that she just adored.

Then Dina got married and began setting up her home. She was forever "needing" things, and there was always something new on the market. Although she had a full-time job and was beginning to raise a family, shopping began to take on a life of its own. She shopped for pots and linen, for clothes and dishes, furnishings, gadgets, jewelry ... Her shopping sprees were so exciting, but they were exhausting!

Then shopping on the Internet became the modus operandi, and Dina was ecstatic! She could shop whenever and wherever she wanted. No more traipsing through stores. No more making arrangements so she could get to the mall before it closed, or taking a day off from her job. Whatever Dina wanted, Dina ordered.

By that time she didn't necessarily **need** what she ordered. She simply enjoyed the excitement of ordering the items, getting them delivered and seeing them in her closet, on her shelf, in her kitchen ... wherever.

< 180 >

After a while, the packages and boxes began to accumulate unopened in the closets, under the bed, in the basement. Dina didn't even bother unwrapping the clothes, or unpacking the boxes. As time went on the purchases began to amass, and Dina found it necessary to find new and more hiding places.

All this time Dina's husband was blissfully unaware of the growing problem. He did not pay the bills nor keep track of their finances. Since he learned in *kollel,* he had accepted other household responsibilities that excluded any monetary concerns.

One day, however, Dina's husband, Mordy, tried to pay with the credit card for an emergency replacement part for the refrigerator, and the charge was declined. Mordy was taken aback and immediately called the credit card company for clarification. They explained that they had already raised the limit on the charge card to $20,000, but the card had nevertheless been "maxed out."

Mordy didn't know there were many more charge cards that they owned that were also maxed out. All he knew for sure was that something was definitely wrong.

When his wife came home from work that day, he asked her for an explanation. Although at first she vehemently denied any knowledge of a problem, it didn't take long for reality to set in. She broke down and cried.

Dina was a shopaholic, an oniomaniac in clinical terms. Her pastime was a real and destructive addiction that had her family on the path to financial disaster.

Mordy and Dina realized they needed help without delay, so when they called me for an appointment, I readily agreed to meet with them. They recounted the events that had led them to my door to seek guidance. I advised Dina to

< 181 >

immediately join one of the support groups for people facing similar issues. Previous experience with predicaments of this nature also indicated a need to put Dina and Mordy in contact with a financial planner who could help them work out a both a budget plan and a payment schedule for their debts. Since Dina had been exhibiting this behavior for a long period of time, I suggested that she seek professional help to work out some personal issues that might be underlying her compulsive behavior. Lastly, I also recommended a course of "spiritual therapy" that would enable the young couple to derive strength and encouragement from Torah and *mitzvos*.

• • •

< 182 >

Relatively speaking, the study of compulsive shopping disorder is fairly new, compared to alcoholism or drug abuse. Nevertheless, more and more evidence is indicating that it is a serious problem and diagnostic criteria have been proposed for inclusion in the Diagnostic and Statistical Manual (DSM).

In truth, we all love to shop – some more than others. It's a favorite pastime of many to spend hours in the mall, buying new clothes, the latest gadgets, or an eye-catching trinket. Moreover, we have become a society that measures social worth by possessions.

Shlomo HaMelech tells us in *Koheles (6:7)*, "Man's wants are never satisfied." Ibn Ezra explains that the soul of man is only sated and content with Torah and *maasim tovim* (good deeds).

Our task is to fulfill the will of the *neshamah*, and man was therefore created with the desires and abilities to live a life of Torah – a life of spirituality. Our sages attest that gratification and happiness are closely linked to the *neshamah*, and it is, in fact, the soul that effects contentment. The Chachmas Koheles cites the Zohar that Hashem looked into the Torah and then created the world, i.e. the Torah establishes the purpose of human existence. Only a life of Torah and *mitzvos* brings man true serenity and a feeling of being complete.

The avid shopper, or one who shops excessively and accumulates "possessions," may not be operating within the spirit of Torah law, but he/she is not clinically a shopaholic. "Oniomania," or shopping addiction, is defined as the demonstration of a profound inability to resist one's impulse to shop despite negative consequences socially, financially, professionally, or maritally. The individual buys more than he/she can afford, buys items that are not needed, and buys them in multiple quantities. For example, the compulsive shopper may buy ten or twenty CDs at a time, or five pairs of the same style shoe in different colors.

< 183 >

Man's life on this earth is characterized as a struggle between the *yetzer hara* (the Evil Inclination) and the *yetzer tov* (the Good Inclination). The task of the *yetzer tov* is to influence us to go in the ways of Torah, to perform the *mitzvos*, and to raise our spiritual level closer to Hashem. The objective of the Evil Inclination, however, is to lure us away from the true path of Torah and to bring about our spiritual downfall.

The Talmud *(Berachos 61a)* comments, "Woe is to me because of my Creator, woe is to me because of my Evil Inclination." Rashi notes that the individual is anguished because if he heeds his inclination he will be accountable to his Creator. If he wrestles with the *yetzer hara*, and tries to avoid submitting to his inclination, he will be plagued with tormenting thoughts.

Men are just as likely to buy compulsively as women; their tastes and habits, though, differ. Female compulsive shoppers buy clothes, shoes, jewelry, cosmetics and gifts for friends, perhaps believing that these will give others a better impression of them. Men are more often "collectors" of things such as electronics, hardware and CDs, but will also buy shoes and clothing. Consciously or subconsciously, some seek greater self-esteem, to fill an inner need, or to buy love. Others shop out of loneliness, depression, or to distract them from uncomfortable feelings.

Compulsive shoppers shop without regard to the economic climate; their addiction is not linked to their financial status. When they are flush, the excessive shopping can be more easily dismissed or hidden. In hard times, though, the impulse to shop becomes an addiction that few can afford.

According to Dr. Donald Black, a psychiatry professor who specializes in obsessive-compulsive disorder, compulsive shopping isn't actually a compulsion; rather it is an impulse-control disorder. Dr. Black explains that a compulsion is a physical or mental behavior used to alleviate an anxiety and

< 184 >

upsetting thought. Compulsive shopping, on the other hand, is not triggered by upsetting thoughts. It is a gratifying impulse to which the compulsive shopper responds. "It's not a lack of willpower that makes them unable to stop shopping," says Dr. Timothy Fong, director of the UCLA Addiction Medicine Clinic, "it's an inability to control their impulses and desires."

HaGaon HaRav Eliyahu Dessler observes that people in this world are preoccupied with possessions, laboring under the false impression that it will bring them true happiness. In reality, though, this hunger for materialism cannot be sated in this world, because it is impossible to satisfy fantasy. Our sages tell us that when a person dies he has not acquired even half of what he desires (*Medrash Rabbah Koheles*).

Studies indicate that as many as 17 million Americans, or more than one in 20, cannot control their urge to shop. Contrary to common thought, men and women are almost equally compulsive buyers (Sanford study 2006). Most shopaholics do not typically refer themselves for counseling. They are generally referred by a law enforcement officer, because many compulsive shoppers end up shoplifting when they can no longer pay for their obsessive purchasing binges; or by a spouse and/or a financial counselor, because they cannot pay their bills, their credit rating is negatively affected, their credit cards are maxed out, they have collection agencies pursuing them for payment, or they are facing bankruptcy.

Generally, the compulsive shopper has a preoccupation with shopping. Making purchases brings a blast of relief from uncomfortable feelings and the tension that has built up from that shopping fixation.

"Rava observed: First the Evil Inclination is called a passer-by, then he is called a guest, and finally he is called a man" (*Succah 52b*). The Vilna Gaon explains that initially the *yetzer hara* is only a thought, an idea that one reflects upon,

< 185 >

but he does not consider acting upon it. If the person briefly disengages himself from the ways of Torah at times, and yields to his weaknesses, the *yetzer hara* becomes a guest in his psyche. As the person moves further away from the ways of Torah the *yetzer hara* takes up residence in his psyche and becomes the *baal habayis* (homeowner). At that point the Evil Inclination is in charge.

Similar to other addictive behaviors, the compulsive shopper engages in this activity in order to escape life, to the point where his behavior takes full control of him/her. In fact, compulsive shopping can be just as addictive and destructive as alcohol or drugs. Brain-imaging studies show that people, even "normal" shoppers, who look forward to buying something exhibit a surge of activity in many of the same pleasure-seeking brain circuits as the alcoholic who is anticipating drinking.

Oniomania usually is cyclical. The addict who is preoccupied with shopping experiences unpleasant feelings of depression, guilt, or boredom. Despite the fact that the compulsive shopper is perfectly aware of what she is doing and is fully cognizant of the financial difficulties she may face, the urge to shop is uncontrollable. The shopping venture is satisfying, rewarding, and enjoyable. After the shopping binge, though, there comes the letdown. The shopaholic is plagued by guilt feelings and remorse over the money that has been wasted and/or the debt that has been incurred. This sends the oniomaniac back to the stores for another "high" of shopping.

The purchases are relegated to the closets, drawers, basements and attics with the tags still attached, often still in the shopping bags. Some compulsive shoppers enter a cycle of buying and returning, but can never return items without buying new ones. Some just give away their purchases, but quickly run out for another shopping spree to replace the items with new ones.

< 186 >

Shifra's Story

I often contemplated the intent of the *pasuk* in *Tehillim* (27:10), "Though my father and mother have forsaken me, Hashem will gather me in," and attributed it to an involuntary abandonment, perhaps the death of one's parents.

I learned otherwise one bright sunny day in July when a local *askan* called me about a teenage girl in the community. Shifra had been thrown out of her house and had nowhere to go. The *askan* pleaded with me to listen to her story so that together we could decide what could be done.

It was difficult to listen to the poignantly sad and disturbing story. Shifra was the oldest of a large family in a mildly dysfunctional home. The deprivation was not only manifest physically; there was also a lack of emotional succor. Neither parent had the capacity to be affectionate or warm and demonstrative. The older children struggled, each in their own way; the younger children were still too naïve to comprehend what they lacked.

Shifra endeavored to retain her composure as she began to explain what had precipitated her expulsion from home.

"In the last few years I would often find myself wandering the aisles of the large neighborhood drugstores and chain stores, checking out the glittering trinkets, colorful cosmetics, array of perfumes, and other small items that caught my eye. First I only bought something when I had a few dollars. Then I got a credit card offer in the mail, and I quickly filled out the form and was approved.

"Voila! I now had my own money to spend. I didn't know what to buy first. Whenever I had the opportunity I would go into the stores and buy whatever intrigued me. Subconsciously I was aware that the more bitter my disappointments were and

< 187 >

the deeper my pain, the more purchases I made. I soon found it difficult to make even the small monthly payments on my credit card bill.

"I borrowed money from my friends; I begged money from others. I had no shame. The emptiness I felt inside of me could only be satisfied with more purchases, more lipsticks and tchotchkes, more baubles and novelty items. I knew I was out of control, but I needed that 'pick-me-up' more.

"The day came when I had no one from whom to borrow or beg anymore. When I walked into the pharmacy that day I knew I didn't have a penny in my pocket, and I was acutely aware that my credit card had been maxed out.

"However, when I strolled the long wide aisles and looked longingly at all the shiny objects beckoning, I realized that no one was around. 'Hmm,' I thought to myself, 'what would happen if I just took some items and surreptitiously hid them under my capacious hoodie? I don't think anyone will notice.'

"And that's exactly what I did. There was a large display of new makeup that had come in and I took the beautiful little cosmetics case that came with a set of eyeshadows, along with three bottles of nail polish. No alarms went off, and nobody came rushing down the aisle to apprehend me. So I reached down to pick up the two tubes of lipstick that were so tempting, and added them to my hidden cache.

"I contemplated taking a bottle of my favorite perfume but decided I would come back the next day wearing something more roomy, perhaps with deep pockets.

"I looked around once more. Nobody seemed to have the slightest interest in my activities, so I casually turned and walked down the aisle to the front of the store and headed for the exit.

< 188 >

"As I walked through the door, I was accosted by the security guard who had been waiting outside for me. I can't believe I was so guileless as not to think of surveillance cameras, but I had been under scrutiny from the moment I pocketed the first item. Due to the high volume of shoplifting, the pharmacy had recently implemented a policy of zero tolerance and had every intention of pressing charges against me.

"I was detained until the police arrived. They took me down to the precinct where I was photographed and fingerprinted and then allowed to make my one phone call."

Shifra began to cry uncontrollably. After a few minutes, when she was able to speak again, she sobbed, "My mother said, 'If you were taken to prison, then stay there. Maybe you'll grow up there and learn how to behave.'"

It was only the hand of Hashem that happened to bring a member of Shomrim into the police precinct just as Shifra was being taken for fingerprinting. His inquiries at the desk brought the *askan* there to post bail.

Indeed, as the *pasuk* in *Tehillim* concludes, "Hashem will gather me in." Shifra will need much *siyata d'shmaya* as she is criminally charged and seeks a home, hopefully one that is nowhere near a prison cell.

● ● ●

< 189 >

Are You a Compulsive Shopper?

- Do you have a closet filled with purchases that still have the tags on them and have never been worn?

- Do you go to the store to buy one pair of shoes but walk out with five?

- Do you buy excessive amounts of items that never get used or that you already have at home?

- Do you spend far beyond your means, putting yourself in massive debt?

- Are you borrowing or stealing money to shop?

- Do you return items to the store out of guilt, feel pressured by being in the store, and then buy other items?

- Do you buy things you see or want, regardless of the cost?

- Are you in the hole financially and maxed out on your credit cards?

- Do you lie about your purchases or how much they cost?

< 190 >

Reasons for Compulsive Shopping:

- Emotional deprivation in childhood

- A compulsion to fill an inner void

- An inability to tolerate negative feelings

- Low self-esteem

- Seeking approval in others

- Lack of impulse control

< 191 >

Help

There are two distinct components of the compulsive shopping disorder that must be focused on.

A therapist would be most effective in analyzing the root cause for the oniomania and addressing the problem.

In addition, these expensive shopping spress often result in an accrued huge credit card balance, with a heavily indebted family that may even be facing bankruptcy. A financial consultant helps guide individuals and their families in planning a budget, creating a payment schedule, and strategizing for the future.

Preventing Shopping Binges:

- Recognize the difference between need and want.

- Destroy all credit cards.

- Pay for purchases by cash or debit card.

- Avoid discount warehouses and other triggers, like favorite stores or Internet sites.

- "Window shop" only after stores have closed, or leave your wallet home.

- Shop with a trusted friend.

- Make shopping lists and only buy what is on the list.

- Allow a 48-hour "cooling-off" period before making any purchase (30 days for major purchases).

- Join a support group.

< 192 >

Spiritual Help

The Mishnah in *Pirkei Avos (4:1)* states, "Who is rich? He who is happy with what he has," i.e. he does not seek or desire more. It would seem, states HaGaon HaRav Eliyahu Schlesinger *shlita*, that personal wealth is not gauged by how much one possesses but rather by how much he feels he is missing. Our sages teach us, "One who has one hundred [dollars] desires two hundred," indicating that man always craves more than he has. Thus, one who is actually "satisfied" with his portion is indeed wealthy.

There are some steps a person can take to diminish or divert his drive to pursue material acquisitions:

- Study books (*sefarim*) that deal with issues of *bitachon*, faith in Hashem.

- Learn to develop an appreciation for the possessions, resources, and blessings that you do have.

- Become involved in charitable acts of lovingkindness, i.e. visiting the sick, and helping poor and underprivileged families.

- Redirect your shopping activities, to experience disciplined spending required for *hachnasas kallah* projects, soup kitchens and the like.

- Pray to Hashem for help to subjugate the intense impulses that drive the overspending.

< 193 >

Food Addiction

< 195 >

Food Addiction

HaGaon HaRav Pinchas HaLevi Horowitz, the Hafla'ah, (1731-1805) posits that the action of eating encompasses two realms. There is the desire of man to sate his physical hunger, but there is also a second sphere in which the consumption of food involves a spiritual factor.

As we know, there are four levels of creation in the world: domeim – the inanimate objects; tzomei'ach – vegetation; chai – living creatures, that is, animals; and medaber – the human being who possesses the power of speech.

Rabbi Horowitz explains that one aspect of tikkun ha'olam – repairing the world – involves the elevation of each creation to a higher plane. Thus, when a person partakes of his food with a divine purpose, he raises that food to a higher level by imbuing it with a spiritual element. In this way, the tzomei'ach – vegetation – is raised to the level of a chai, so to speak, and achieves its higher root in the world.

< 197 >

Kaylie's Story

Following one of my presentations on eating disorders, a young woman approached me outside the auditorium. She explained that she had been bingeing for the past five years and was desperately seeking help. After listening to me speak she felt that I would be able to help her. I gave her my contact information, and we subsequently set up an appointment. Her story is not extraordinary, but it is shocking to the uninitiated.

Kaylie presented as an upbeat, happy-go-lucky girl who didn't have a care in the world. When she arrived at my office, she seemed anxious to speak.

"Rabbi Goldwasser," she burst out, "I wish I could lose weight and I could get better. I have a sister who is stick-skinny and she eats so so much. How does she do it? She's so lucky!"

Kaylie's account was fraught with the red flags that indicate a problem, and her façade of self-confidence and high spirits slowly crumbled as she related the events associated with her addiction to food.

> "I don't know what is wrong with me. This morning, for example, I was all bloated. I really felt yuk – even though I didn't binge at night. That's because I really wasn't feeling good yesterday and I was petrified. Today I wasn't hungry at all but I ate anyway. I don't really want to eat, but something inside forces me to do it. It's only 2:00 in the afternoon and I've already eaten a generous portion of chocolate mousse cake and two bagels in the morning, with some more cake and three bagels for an early lunch."

Kaylie was the fifth of twelve children. They did not live in

< 198 >

a big house, and Kaylie often found that she lacked her "space." Five siblings were already happily married, one younger than she. At twenty-three, Kaylie wanted very much to join her friends in matrimonial bliss, but so far she had not met "Mr. Right." Her desperation to leave home was clear in her voice.

> "Regarding marriage, why can't I believe that everything will be OK ... I do try to dream and think of good things, but nothing has happened yet so I am discouraged."

She stated that she really loved her mother, but her description depicted a difficult relationship with her. Her mother was a stern, no-nonsense woman who was more of a judgmental sort. She did not tolerate weakness or permissiveness and ran a tight ship. Kaylie seemed to have many disagreements with her mother on multiple issues from her clothing to helping at home and everything in between. Those invariably led to big-time bingeing.

> "I've been eating a lot. An abnormal amount, even though my stomach is full – so full that it hurts. But I still keep eating. I'm stuffed, but my mouth is watering and wants more and more. I never seem to be satiated. I've also been chewing and spitting out – it's absolutely disgusting. I am put off from myself! This is *gehennom!*"

Shabbos was especially trying for Kaylie. She didn't like to eat/binge in front of the Shabbos guests who invariably visited their home. She admitted,

> "When I binge I only eat bad foods, so I know I'm lacking in a lot of nutrients. Thursday I wasn't feeling good; I was a little dizzy. Friday morning I started with a bowl of cereal and

< 199 >

juice. A half hour later I had two pieces of cake
and two little cheesecakes. Then I had two
fruit roll-ups. It was another messed up day!
I had lots of challah in the afternoon before
candle lighting. Then afterwards, I just couldn't
wait for Kiddush, and I had another generous
helping of chocolate cake and cheesecake. At
the table I only ate one bite of fish, a bowl of
soup, and one bite of chicken."

Kaylie began to cry as she described instances of family
infighting that had been traumatic. Replays of similar
occurrences and abuse only served as triggers for Kaylie's
unhappiness and depression. This fed into her insecurity and
brought to the fore many hashkafic questions that she could
not handle. "It's unbearable," she sobbed. "The pain is so
agonizing."

Kaylie had developed a strong love-hate relationship with
food. Living in a small community out of town, she had no one
with whom she felt comfortable discussing her problem.

She couldn't stop eating, and then would regret every bite
of food she had ingested. At the table she would nibble at her
food, but when no one was home, or late at night she would
raid the refrigerator. Her weight would yo-yo up and down
and her mood was relevant to whether she fit into her clothing
that day.

Although she put on a great face on the outside, Kaylie
was miserable inside. She was self-loathing, had no self-esteem
to speak of, was worried about her relationship with Hashem,
and was afraid for her future wellbeing.

● ● ●

< 200 >

The Chazon Ish once remarked to a colleague that he felt absolutely no different before ingesting food or after eating. If he was presented with food by family members he assumed that he had not yet eaten his meal *(Sefer Pe'er HaDor, Vol. III)*.

Until recently, obesity has been attributed to various factors such as genetics, lack of exercise, and a lack of ability to diet and/or practice portion control. However, studies now seem to indicate that compulsive overeating is driven by a food addiction. It is similar to other substance dependencies, and people who are addicted to food tend to mimic the characteristics of addictive behavior. Studies have shown that many of the brain changes seen in various forms of addiction are also reported in people who overeat. Research is also indicating that a constant pattern of overeating stimulates a normally dormant metabolic response in the hypothalamus region of the brain. The reaction causes increased levels of overeating, generating a vicious cycle that becomes difficult to break.

A clinical psychology doctoral student at the Yale Rudd Center for Food Policy and Obesity indicated that certain foods – especially those containing lots of sugar, salt or fat – can activate the same brain receptors that are triggered by addictive drugs and take control.

Most importantly, similar to drug addiction, for example, overeating and obesity are compelled by physical, mental and emotional cravings and repeated exposure to trigger foods.

Although such people tend to be overweight, by and large, "normal weight" people can be addicted to food as well.

< 201 >

Sophie's Story

Food – unlike alcohol or drugs – is essential to survival and most people eat a few times every day. People keep fresh food in their refrigerator, have canned goods in their pantry, or they can call any one of the local eateries for a ready-cooked meal. In this aspect, it is more difficult for the food addict to successfully control his cravings, simply because of the absolute availability of the addictive substance. In fact, in my twenty-five years of experience working in the field of eating disorders, I have come to see that food addiction is sometimes more formidable and intense than other addictions.

Sophie, a native of Los Angeles, had come to New York to study in seminary. She was a capable young woman who did well in her studies. She generally did volunteer work with mothers who had newborns and were overwhelmed with familial obligations. Although reticent by nature, Sophie demonstrated an innate ability to relate to young children. She was gentle, funny and playful, and well-liked by everyone who met her.

Sophie's wonderful reputation preceded her. When she finished seminary, she was immediately hired by one of the top schools in the area as a first grade teacher. The students absolutely adored Sophie. The parents were delighted that their children were so happy in the classroom and noted their academic progress in class with deep satisfaction. The staff was especially pleased with Sophie's performance, and pleased that their decision to hire her had been on the mark.

Sophie, personally, was glad that she had been offered this wonderful position, because she would never have applied on her own to this particular school. Sophie, in fact, had some personal issues which hampered her in many ways. Sophie had one sibling, a brother, and their childhood had been trying. They had grown up with detached and unloving parents, and

< 202 >

were conditioned to believe that they were of little value in themselves. Sophie, especially, was more socially withdrawn, had an inability to accept compliments, and lacked self-confidence. She did not contribute much to conversations and kept her opinions to herself, in order to avoid any possibility of rejection or derision.

Once she left home, Sophie had gradually made a few friends but remained reserved and rented her own apartment. She didn't expect much out of life for herself and was resigned to the unlikeliness of finding a "good" *shidduch*. Nevertheless, for the first few months in her new job Sophie was content, in her comfort zone, in the company of the non-judgmental young children.

After a few months, though, Sophie became ill at ease with her job performance, agonized about her lesson plans, and was reluctant to trust her judgment. She brooded over any mistake she had made during the school day, and questioned her accomplishments. As her anxiety and apprehension increased, food became a major companion. At the end of an evening at home, she would notice that she had eaten her way through an entire extra-large bag of potato chips, or had finished a half-gallon container of ice cream instead of the three spoonfuls she had originally set out to eat. Soon, she wasn't buying one quarter of chicken for supper, but two or three quarters with a generous helping of side dishes.

Sophie realized she was feeling a little depressed and eating for comfort, but was not too concerned. She rationalized that, as in the past, she would eventually regain her mental equilibrium and allay her negative thoughts. She hoped that her dependency on food would dissipate as well.

One day, however, Sophie did something very unusual during the school day. As she did every day, Sophie prepared an afternoon snack of cookies and milk for her class in the small

< 203 >

kitchenette next door. Sometimes, if she was hungry, she would grab a cookie for herself. That afternoon, though, as Sophie prepared the snacks for the class, she wolfed down an entire package of cookies herself. What is more, she barely took the time to chew the cookies and enjoy them; she just stuffed them down her throat until the entire bag was empty. Then, realizing the children were waiting for her, she quickly distributed the cookies and milk and returned to the kitchenette to finish off the cookies left over in the second bag.

Initially flabbergasted by what had happened, Sophie felt sick to her stomach. By the time she got to the grocery store later that evening though, to replace the bag of cookies she had demolished, Sophie bought **two** double packages, one for her personal consumption.

Sophie began to develop an obsession for food and about food. All she could think about was food. She was always shopping for food, planning her meals or ordering food from take-out. She would eat loaves of bread, bowls of rice, an entire ice cream cake, or munch her way through bags of snacks until she fell asleep late at night from sheer exhaustion.

By the time Sophie called me she was in the throes of a full-blown eating disorder. Her overeating had accelerated way out of control. The increased stress on Sophie's body was wreaking havoc on her wellbeing; Sophie was experiencing dizzy spells and an irregular heart rate. She was frightened out of her wits.

I listened to Sophie's story and gave her advice and several practical suggestions. Nevertheless, I cautioned her, it was really important that she come in to see me in person so that we could properly address her problem. Sophie was reluctant to do so. She was embarrassed to meet me because she had put on so much weight.

Sophie continued to call me over the next few months but

< 204 >

her situation deteriorated. She was caught in the vicious cycle of using food to cope with her feelings of guilt, shame and unworthiness, which only intensified the compulsion. There were times when Sophie called and just sobbed painfully over the phone, unable to articulate her torment. She stopped going out with the few friends she had, or attending *simchas*, fearful of making a spectacle of herself in public. In fact, for all intents and purposes, she had become a recluse; her only excursions were to school and food shopping.

Sophie's moment of truth was not a pretty picture. Sophie realized that she had reached an all-time low. Once Sophie had reached her body's capacity to retain food, she would be in excruciating pain. Nevertheless, her craving for food was so intense that she would chew the food without swallowing it, spit it out, and then put the masticated food back into her mouth to "feed" her dependency.

In addition, Sophie's "habit" had become very expensive and her financial situation was precarious.

When Sophie called that day she was desperate and ready to meet with me. Sophie was a bright, intelligent young woman and expressed a sincere desire to regain her health and mental equilibrium.

I worked with Sophie for close to nine months, structuring a healthy eating plan, developing stress management techniques and coordinating intensive counseling therapy. It was vital to shift Sophie's attention away from food and refocus her on productive physical and spiritual activities.

We were making very slow but steady progress, and I was hopeful that Sophie's status would normalize to the point where she could be classified as a recovered addict. Unfortunately, this has not been the case to date. Sophie has been in and out of the hospital for the last two years for various medical issues

< 205 >

that have arisen as a result of her compulsive eating disorder. It seems that Sophie's resistance to change is impeding her recovery.

The Talmud (*Avodah Zarah 17a*) relates that R' Elazar ben Dordaya had transgressed every *aveirah* in the world. Once he met up with a woman of ill repute who expelled her breath and said to him, "Just like this breath of air cannot return to its original place, so too Elazar ben Dordaya will not be able to return in repentance."

R' Elazar sat between the mountains and hills and cried out, "Plead for mercy for me that my *teshuvah* should be accepted." They answered him, "Before we could pray for you we have to pray for ourselves."

He called to the heaven and earth, "Please pray for mercy for me," and they too answered, "Before we could pray for you we have to pray for ourselves."

He ran to the sun and moon, "Please pray for mercy for me," and they replied, "We can be destroyed because of these sins. Before we could pray for you we have to pray for ourselves."

He cried out to the stars and constellations, "Please pray for me that my *teshuvah* should be accepted." The stars and constellations said, "How can we pray for you? We need to pray for ourselves that we should not be harmed."

Finally R' Elazar ben Dordaya realized that he could only count on himself; the power to change and do *teshuvah* resided within him. He put his head between his knees and wept so violently that his *neshamah* departed. At that moment a *bas kol* (Heavenly Voice) proclaimed: R' Elazar ben Dordaya has acquired a place in *olam haba* (the World-to-Come).

< 206 >

The Ya'aras Dvash comments that first he went to the mountains, because he identified with that environment. He then approached the heaven and earth – which represent the contrast between spiritual and earthly components of this world – because he had not been able to conquer his *yetzer*, Evil Inclination. He ran to the stars because he wanted to blame his fate on his horoscope and the astrological sign under which he had been born. He wanted to assign culpability for the transgressions in his life to others, until he ultimately understood that he alone was capable of effecting change and the power of *teshuvah* rested entirely in his own hands!

• • •

< 207 >

The Rambam *(Hilchos Dei'os 4:15)* notes that many illnesses are brought about by eating foods that are harmful for one's health or because one has gorged himself, even on healthy food. A physician who is concerned about his patient's health and wellbeing, writes the Rambam in *Shemone Perakim*, should be exacting about the patient's diet. He asserts that overindulgence in food and drink can negatively affect a person's behaviors and character traits.

These principles are supported in *Proverbs (21:23)* where Shlomo HaMelech writes, "*Shomer piv ul'shono shomer mitzaros nafsho* – one who guards his mouth and tongue guards his soul from troubles." Our sages explain this to mean that if a person guards his mouth from eating foods that are not good, or from overindulging, and guards his tongue from speaking improperly, he will be shielded from distress and anguish.

Eating nourishes the body and is generally a pleasurable and satisfying experience that is a natural part of our lives, as we learn in *Koheles (9:7)*, "Go and eat your bread with joy ...." In fact, food is an important component of many events and special occasions, including Shabbos and Yom Tov. Many of us have sometimes even experienced the feeling of having eaten more than we should have.

Pressures of work, a lack of energy, feelings of boredom or loneliness can often upset an otherwise well-adjusted lifestyle. In this context, people turn to food for comfort to avoid or suppress negative emotions, or to fill a need for affection. It leaves one with a feeling of numbness which disassociates him/her from his feelings. They are usually aware that their eating is out of control, but they need the food to fill an internal void and to help them cope with daily stresses in their lives.

Compulsive overeaters consistently eat without control, followed by intense feelings of shame about their behavior and its effects (real or perceived) on their body image. Issues of

< 208 >

powerlessness, guilt and failure are common among individuals with a food addiction. The more weight they gain, the harder they try to diet. They become obsessed with weight loss, instead of focusing on the cause of their weight gain – the compulsive overeating. The deprivation of the foods they enjoy creates a stronger craving for them, and that usually leads to more overeating. This develops into a repetitive tormented cycle of negative feelings that are soothed with food. The suffering individual becomes entangled in a war with his/her own body.

There is an incontrovertible connection between human emotions, the brain and the stomach. As with all eating disorders, a common component is the presence of low self-esteem. Our society has fostered an attitude that associates one's inherent worth with control of one's weight. The reverse – failure – results in self-censure and feelings of humiliation.

The antithesis of compulsive overeating is anorexia, which is self-imposed starvation. Rather than losing control and becoming addicted to food, the anorexic takes control of his/her food intake and weight in a life where he/she otherwise feels powerless, guilt and failure. The causal feelings and issues underlying both disorders are similar; it is the response of the individual that differs.

< 209 >

Peninah's Story

Peninah was a typical, yet unassuming, eighth grader and a straight-A student. Although she was shy, she had a few good friends with whom she was always on the phone. She had the usual heavy load of homework and tests that she breezed through. She loved listening to music and reading, was active in the G.O., participated in all the school projects, and was well known for her *lev tov* (good heart).

Her parents took pleasure in her achievements. And why not? Although they noticed her diffidence – she would sometimes turn red with embarrassment when accepting a compliment – they reckoned she would eventually mature and become more comfortable in her own skin. In fact, they would proudly say, "We are so happy that you are like your older sister, Miriam." The teachers made that comparison as well.

Having recently reached her *bas mitzvah*, and keenly interested in working with special needs children, Peninah had begun to commit an allotted amount of her free hours to help with these children. No one paid much attention, though, to the fact that her *chesed* always coincided with mealtimes. Peninah would respectfully, but casually, request to either eat her meal earlier or later than the family.

Eventually, though, Peninah's weight loss became very obvious. Her clothes were hanging on her, and her features were gaunt. Her luster was gone, and her hair hung limply around her face. When questioned by her parents, she nonchalantly dismissed their concerns, attributing her weight loss to "a teenager thing" and lack of sleep. Reassured that their daughter was every parent's dream, they failed to notice the warning signs of Peninah's entanglement with the world of eating disorders.

Ultimately her weight loss could no longer be explained

< 210 >

that easily, and Peninah was taken to the family doctor who immediately recognized that Peninah was seriously ill. He suggested that they contact me and arrange an appointment. I met first with the parents and then with Peninah herself. The results of the blood work clearly indicated that the disease was already making severe inroads physically, and her condition was deteriorating. Unquestionably, this precious young *nefesh* needed help.

I spoke with Peninah for a couple of hours and discovered that she had been secretly restricting her diet and purging for over a year. Intense issues of low self-esteem surfaced, exacerbated by complex family dynamics and phobias.

I explained to Peninah and the family the importance of a treatment plan and helped them implement it. Initially, we saw Peninah making progress, but then there were some setbacks and Peninah began to backslide quickly.

She became so ill, she had to be rushed to the hospital. I immediately went to visit her. However, nothing prepared me for Peninah's shocking request, after I had sat down.

"I know the Rav for about two months now. I have a request of you which I cannot address to anyone else. Is that okay?"

"Please feel free to ask me anything you need," I calmly assured her.

"But please don't be upset with me," she said to me.

I could not imagine what would offend me, and I said, "Ask what you like."

With tears in her eyes she told me that she felt her time in this world was up and she wanted me to recite the *viduy* with her.

< 211 >

I was thunderstruck. Speechless, I sat there in disbelief, wondering how Peninah had ever reached such a nadir. I was listening to a twelve-year-old girl with the greatest potential, who had every opportunity in the world available to her, who thought her life was over.

Finally, with great effort, I said, "I will do anything possible that I can for you. But I have a different suggestion. Instead of saying *viduy* we could recite the Shalah's *tefillah* for a *refuah shleimah* and some *Tehillim*.

Peninah firmly replied, "Rav, it's okay. I'm not afraid to say *viduy*. It would be easier for me if I didn't have to live anymore. The struggle and the guilt feelings are too much for me. My whole *neshamah* is in pain," and she began to cry bitterly.

I had already opened my *Tehillim*, and without a second's delay, I began to recite the chapter. I continued, without pausing, and finally I saw, out of the corner of my eye, that Peninah was also saying that chapter of *Tehillim*.

I continued to sit with Peninah for hours, talking, listening, and giving *chizuk* (encouragement and inspiration) until I felt that Peninah had turned the corner.

Although I have witnessed hundreds of very difficult and agonizing struggles, none is as heartbreaking as the recollection of the searing pain of a young girl requesting me to recite the *viduy* with her. *Hashem yerachem* (may Hashem have mercy).

• • •

< 212 >

Are You Addicted?

- Do you have a lack of self-control when it comes to food?

  o Eating rapidly
  o Eating large amounts of food when not physically hungry
  o Eating until you feel uncomfortably full
  o Eating more food, and for a longer time, than you had planned to at first

- Do you associate food with a sense of pleasure and/or comfort and are unable to stop using food to create that feeling?

- Do you hide the food or eat in private?

- Do you feel depressed, disgusted or guilty after overeating?

- Do your emotions cause you to eat?

- Do you have a history of marked weight fluctuation?

- Do you continue to overeat, despite being aware of the consequences?

- Have you tried unsuccessfully to cut down on or control your eating?

< 213 >

Help

The Talmud states *(Gittin 70a)*, "If your meal gives you pleasure, take your hand away from it and do not overindulge." HaGaon HaRav Shlomo Zalman Braun in the *Sefer Sha'ar Metzuyanim B'Halacha* notes that the Talmud doesn't say that one should leave the table, rather that he should take away his hand. The author explains that one should not keep on rapidly spooning the food in his mouth, but he should practice restraint, partaking of his food with forethought and good sense.

In general, support programs, cognitive behavioral therapy, as well as a consultation with a nutritionist or eating disorder specialist are recommended for the treatment of food addictions.

Some tips that are helpful include:

- Developing a clear plan of eating

- Being aware which foods trigger an eating binge and eliminating them

- Being aware which situations trigger cravings and/or an eating binge and avoiding them

- Learning stress management techniques

- Building self-esteem and interpersonal skills

- Developing hobbies and interests that do not focus on food

< 214 >

Spiritual Help

The Torah recounts *(Bereishis, 3)* that Adam sinned and, contrary to the command of Hashem, partook of the fruit from the *eitz hada'as* (Tree of Knowledge). In his explanation for succumbing to temptation, Adam states, "The woman whom You gave to be with me – she gave me of the tree, and I eat."

Rav Abba bar Kahana (Midrashic sage) notes that Adam didn't say "I ate" (in the past tense), but used the present tense, "I eat," meaning, "I have eaten from the forbidden fruit and I will continue to eat."

The Kotzker Rebbe remarks on the ostensible arrogance of Adam towards his Creator. It would be comparable to someone caught red-handed stealing who argues, "I stole this, but I will continue to steal from others."

The Kotzker explains that Adam's defense was actually a statement that reflected a deeper insight into his own psyche. Adam was able to identify his own vulnerability and weakness; he was aware that he was totally under the influence of the Evil Inclination, at the present. He understood that at this point in time it was probable that he would repeat his transgression and eat from the forbidden fruit again.

Often a person will rationalize and minimize his wrongdoings, even to himself. Once behaviors and conduct have become habitual they are difficult to change. It is easier to steer clear of any introspection than to contemplate one's actions and consider their implications.

An individual who has engaged in soul-searching and achieved a sense of self-awareness will ultimately succeed. Understanding one's own nature, abilities and limitations, and having an insight into one's personality and individuality

< 215 >

is basic for the development of character. It is a powerful catalyst for change.

For those wishing additional information and a greater understanding of eating disorders, please refer to my book, *Starving Souls* (Ktav Publishing).

< 216 >

The Addictive Relationship

< 217 >

No examination of the subject of addictions can be complete without discussing addictive relationships. It must be understood at the outset that addictions are not limited to substances. An individual who is compulsively obsessed with an activity, an object or a behavior that gives him/her pleasure is considered to be addicted.

Research indicates that physical addiction to chemicals and psychological dependency on activities, such as gambling or relationships, share many common characteristics.

The addictive relationship consumes the person's life. All of his/her time, energy and hopes are invested in the relationship, often to the detriment of work or other relationships.

The addictive relationship is usually not reciprocal. This may be because the other party is not available, i.e. committed to someone else, is not interested in the relationship, or is emotionally unavailable.

The addicted individual will offer various reasons for continuing the relationship, and/or will deny his predicament.

Despite the pain the relationship often causes, the addicted individual is unable to withdraw, even if he/she wants to do so.

Thinking about ending the relationship generates extreme feelings of anxiety and fear.

When the relationship does end, the addicted individual suffers withdrawal symptoms, including depression and sleeplessness.

Analyses of the addictive relationship reveal that the affinity takes two forms.

< 218 >

In one, the relationship is an imagined one, where the individual has an "attachment hunger." Such an individual feel a sense of incompleteness, emptiness and sadness when not in a relationship and believes that the relationship will fulfill him and relieve his despair. He/she seeks love, attention and security, rather than a shared experience. This individual is addicted to verifying his/her appeal and acceptance even by an uninterested person.

Sometimes, though, the two parties in the relationship are addicted to each other. There are intense feelings of infatuation, jealousy and possessiveness. They are unable to endure separation and have limited or no social contact outside of the relationship. Each party is motivated by his/her own need for security, with little common ground or shared appreciation for each other.

Any plan for addiction recovery is predicated on the individual's commitment to be completely honest with himself and others.

The difficulty in being honest is indubitable. Prevarication and deceptiveness have become an integral part of the addict's life, to the extent that he no longer has the ability to identify the truth. In addition, the addict fears the consequences of honesty, which will result in the abdication of a familiar and comfortable part of himself.

Truth be told, however, if the addict persists in deceiving himself/herself about the severity of his addiction, it is unlikely that any meaningful action will be taken to overcome the addiction.

As has been noted throughout the book, the first step towards recovery is the recognition and acknowledgement that one is entangled in an addictive relationship.

< 219 >

Once the individual has accepted his addiction, he must be willing to confront the unhealthy aspects of his behavior and face his shortcomings.

The addicted individual will need to analyze what is motivating the addiction.

Counseling is usually recommended to help the addicted individual because

• he/she is unable to successfully end the relationship.

• he/she recognizes a destructive pattern of seeking relationships that are not reciprocated.

• he/she needs help in reclaiming their "self."

• he/she needs guidance in processing and healing the issues that impelled the addictive relationship.

• he/she must learn what a healthy relationship is.

The paradigm of *ahavah* (love) is presented in *Ethics of Our Fathers (5:19)*, "Any love that depends on a specific cause, when that cause is gone the love is gone; but if it does not depend on a specific cause, it will never cease. What love depended upon a specific cause? The love of Amnon for Tamar. And what did not depend upon a specific cause? The love of Dovid and Yonasan."

It is noteworthy that the *ahavah* is described in the Mishnah as **depending** on a certain consideration, rather than **resulting** from a specific consideration. The relationship of Amnon and Tamar was corrupted by the excessive consideration of external factors. In contrast, the relationship of Dovid and Yonasan manifested no such consideration. They each only cared about the welfare of the other, with no concern for their own personal satisfaction.

< 220 >

It is, in fact, possible that the *ahavah* may initially be fostered because of a particular factor, but ultimately the relationship must be nurtured and cultivated so that it is no longer dependent on that external aspect.

Rabbeinu Yonah explains that *ahavah* based on external factors is, in effect, selfish, and motivated solely by self-interest. It is an ephemeral love that disappears as soon as the egotism is removed. Thus, once Amnon's obsession was gratified, he hated Tamar more than he initially loved her.

The Rambam differentiates between three forms of *ahavah*. There is the love that is beneficial for both parties, like business partners who have a functional relationship. The second is a love that offers comfort or security. The third, and highest form of *ahavah*, is one that is based on a joint dedication and desire to do good. Such an *ahavah* is not based on external factors, i.e. "does not depend upon a specific cause," and is truly a wholesome *ahavah*.

The Meshech Chachmah analyzes the two terms *ahavah* and *cheshek*, love and desire. He observes that *ahavah* is a more disciplined emotion, whereas *cheshek* has a tendency to get out of control. The disparity of these two emotions may be what differentiates an addictive relationship from a healthy one.

The Jewish idea of marriage is a complementary relationship. The Torah tells us *(Bereishis 1:27)*, "Male and female He created them." Originally man and woman were created as an androgynous unit, and then separated into two separate entities. Their natural tendency is to be one, and marriage is the unification of the two halves into one complete entity.

Marriage, ideally, is based on an altruistic, selfless love. A relationship that is built on a selfish *ahavah* is one that is conditional. In such a situation, each partner seeks to have

< 221 >

his/her own needs met; the relationship is completely self-interested.

A healthy relationship consists of give-and-take. Our sages state *(Derech Eretz Zuta, 2)* that if one wants to love his fellow man then he should do something for his benefit. The *Orchas Tzaddikim* explains that it is the act of doing something for another person that evokes feelings of *ahavah* for the other person. That is to say that love is not based on the satisfaction that one obtains from the relationship; rather, it is fostered by the effort and devotion one expends for the relationship.

When such commitment to the relationship is lacking, an unwholesome co-dependence develops, whereby one partner needs the other to compensate for his inadequacies. This is often the underpinning of an addictive relationship.

< 222 >

The Twelve Step Spiritual Program for Addictions

< 223 >

The Twelve Step
Spiritual Program For Addictions

The following Twelve Step Program was developed exclusively by the author and represents a framework of Torah hashkafa that one needs to integrate into his/her mindset in pursuit of a life of contentment, fulfillment, and success. Each step consists of the core principle, cited verbatim as originally presented by the Alcoholics Anonymous organization. It is followed by a unique and penetrating interpretation of each step from a distinctive Torah perspective that will be helpful in promoting spiritual growth and shielding every individual from the negative forces that surround us in our everyday world.

Step One

We admitted we were powerless over our addiction — that our lives had become unmanageable.

> The Rambam in *Hilchos Teshuvah* establishes the very basic outline of *teshuvah* which consists of four key elements, the first and foremost being recognizing that one has committed a sin, *hakaras hachet*. (That is followed by *viduy*, admitting that one has committed a sin; *azivas hachet*, abandoning the sin; and *kabbalah al ha'asid*, making a firm commitment never to commit the sin again.)

> HaGaon HaRav Eliyahu Dessler writes that every person has a *nekudas habechirah* – a point within him that is conflicted between the Good Inclination and the Evil Inclination. He explains this by presenting the concept of a battlefield, where the actual fighting only takes place in a limited area, i.e. the battlefront. The territory

< 224 >

behind the front on each side is in the respective control of each army and remains uninvolved in battle.

Similarly, says Rav Dessler, each individual's free will *(bechirah)* is only invoked at the battlefront, at that point where the power of good and evil are equally balanced. The purpose of the Evil Inclination is to challenge each person's efforts to elevate himself spiritually. When a person makes the conscious decision to do good, then he raises his spiritual level. Simultaneously, his *nekudas habechirah,* or the line of battle, is moved. That is to say, when a person has conquered his *yetzer hara* (Evil Inclination) in a particular conflict, then that area is annexed to **his** territory, so to speak.

Once someone who is addicted has succumbed to his substance of choice, by constantly making negative choices, he has given in to his inclination, and his *nekudas habechirah* has shifted. His freedom of choice has been compromised because it is more difficult for him to distinguish between the good and the bad. In fact, his judgment is so impaired that he can no longer even identify the prohibition he has breached.

< 225 >

Step Two

Came to believe that a Power greater than ourselves could restore us to sanity.

The Talmud *(Kiddushin 30b)* states, "The *yetzer hara* within the person renews itself each day and wants to destroy him; were it not for Hashem's help he would never be able to overcome him." We find the same statement with a slight variation in *Succah (52b)* which says that the *yetzer hara* "strengthens" itself. These are not, in fact, contradictory concepts; rather the *yetzer hara* wishes to destroy a person in any way possible and adapts itself accordingly.

When the *yetzer hara* is trying to lure a new victim into its trap, it needs to be creative. The Evil Inclination "renews" itself each day by thinking of new strategies and schemes that will succeed in ensnaring the individual. For those who have already become entrapped in the *yetzer hara's* web, the Evil Inclination "strengthens" itself in order to intensify its appeal, tapping deeper into the individual's Achilles' heel, and further severing his relationship with Hashem.

It is for this reason, in fact, that we need Hashem's help in defeating the *yetzer hara*. Nevertheless, explains the Chofetz Chaim, this does not exempt man from exerting every effort, investing his own potential and resourcefulness, in order to fight the *yetzer hara*. If he does so, then Hashem will surely help him.

We ask Hashem *(Tehillim 27:11)*, "Instruct me, Hashem, in Your way and lead me on

< 226 >

the path of uprightness." The Maharam M'Brod explains there are many roads that lead to Hashem. Some are dangerous and present obstacles. Others are circuitous. We pray to Hashem every day, "Do not let me be misled by my improper choices as in the past. Show me Your way; lead me in the direct, straight path to *olam haba.*"

This is similar to the request, "Teach me, Hashem, the way of Your statutes" *(Tehillim 119:33).* Often times a person instinctively knows the correct path to walk in life, however he lacks the self-discipline and control to follow the straight and narrow. David HaMelech entreats Hashem, let me know Your ways –let me be privileged to learn the Torah so that I can appreciate it and understand the significance of the *mitzvos* and their ultimate purpose. Then help me and guide me, even when I may be contrary and unwilling.

< 227 >

Step Three

Made a decision to turn our will and our lives over to the care of G-d as we understood Him.

Twice a day, in the morning and before we go to sleep, we recite the *Adon Olam* prayer, referring to Hashem as the Master of the Universe Who is eternal, unique and strong. Moreover, we entrust our soul in His Hand, that is to say that we recognize that we are in Hashem's care during the day and through the night. HaGaon HaRav Samson Raphael Hirsch points out that while *Adon Olam* speaks of the omnipotence of Hashem, it also refers to Him in a very personal way, "*veHu Keli* – He is my G-d."

We conclude the *Adon Olam*, "Hashem is with me, I shall not fear." This expresses our trust, *bitachon*, that we have nothing to fear. The real proof of *bitachon* in Hashem is that one is unafraid. This is reminiscent of the words of *Tehillim (23:4)*, "Though I walk in the valley overshadowed by death, I will fear no evil for You are with me, Hashem …"

In the afternoon Shabbos prayer we say, "Avraham would rejoice, Yitzchak would exult..." The Beis Yosef and the Ohr HaChaim say that this makes reference to the *Akeidah* (the binding of Yitzchak). HaGaon Rav Elazar Menachem Mann Shach expounds that this teaches us that one should be jubilant and joyful even in times of distress and crisis.

The Vilna Gaon writes that one who is a *ba'al bitachon* – trusts in Hashem – is the reverse of

< 228 >

one who is a *ba'al taavah* – ruled by his desires. Furthermore, states the Gaon, one who has committed serious transgressions but remains a *ba'al bitachon* is greater than one who is involved in Torah learning and the performance of good deeds but lacks *bitachon*.

The Mishnah in *Avos (2:4)* states, "Make His will as if it were your own will, so that He will treat your will as if it were His will." The Sfas Emes explains that if one establishes Hashem's will – i.e. the Torah and the *mitzvos* – as his mainstay, he becomes rooted and balanced. It also creates a reciprocal relationship between Hashem and man, whereby Hashem responds in kind to man's adherence to Torah and *mitzvos*. In a similar vein, the Ari HaKadosh states that if one will resolve to have no other will than to follow the *ratzon Hashem*, then Hashem will, measure for measure *(middah k'neged middah)*, grant the *ratzon* of the individual.

< 229 >

Step Four

Made a searching and fearless moral inventory of ourselves.

The Hebrew word for an accounting of the soul is *cheshbon hanefesh*. The root word of *cheshbon* is *chashuv* – important. Taking inventory of our actions and character traits is an essential tool for self-improvement. It enables one to assess where he is and what needs to be done in order for him/her to move forward.

HaGaon HaRav Yechezkel Levenstein (1884-1974), *mashgiach* of Mir and Ponovezh, suggests that aside from its practical relevance in one's spiritual life in this world, making a *cheshbon hanefesh* is meritorious after 120 years, at the time of Heavenly Judgment.

R' Moshe Chaim Luzzatto, writes in his *Mesilas Yesharim*, "... man should observe all of his actions and his ways so he should not become accustomed to bad habits, negative traits, or sin ... a person should carefully examine his ways and his deeds, to weigh them daily like the merchants who weigh and evaluate their gems constantly. He should set aside specific times and hours for this accounting ..."

The *Mesilas Yesharim* continues that if one will conduct himself in this manner he will be able to correct his ways, as it says *(Eichah 3:40)*, "Let us search and examine our ways and return to Hashem."

A daily accounting of the soul gives a person

< 230 >

the opportunity and wherewithal to review and track his actions of the day when he can still recall them. This forestalls procrastination and facilitates the implementation of the *teshuvah* process.

This can be compared to one who inadvertently spills black dye all over the floor of his house. If he acts quickly and promptly washes away the dye, he will avoid major damage to his floor. If he is slow to respond, allowing the pigment to seep into the floor, it will be very difficult, if not impossible, to rectify the situation.

Rabbi Nachman of Breslov heartens us: If one believes that it is possible to destroy, one must also believe that it is feasible to repair. This recalls the *pasuk* in *Mishlei (24:16)*, "Though the righteous one may fall seven times, he will arise." If a person will instigate the process of *cheshbon hanefesh*, he will be able to execute the steps of *teshuvah* and rise above his challenges, no matter how far he has fallen.

< 231 >

Step Five

Admitted to G-d, to ourselves, and to another human being the exact nature of our wrongs.

As we mentioned, *teshuvah* is comprised of four basic components. The first is *hakaras hachet* – recognition of the sin – discussed earlier. The second is *viduy* – admitting that one has done a sin.

The Rambam *(Hilchos Teshuvah 1:1)* writes that if one transgresses one of the Torah's commandments (positive or negative), whether intentionally or inadvertently, he is obligated to confess his sin as part of his *teshuvah*. This is mandated by the Torah *(Bamidbar 5:6-7)* and is known as *viduy*. According to the Rambam this constitutes the essence of *teshuvah*.

How does one confess: He says, "Please, Hashem, I have sinned, trespassed and rebelled before You, and I have done such and such. I regret and I am shamed by what I have done, and I will try to never repeat it."

Confession, the act of articulating one's feelings of repentance and expressing them aloud, makes one's misdeeds and offenses more real. The verbal confession makes it harder to withdraw; it brings the inner thoughts and emotions from within out into the open. It is a humbling experience that makes it easier for the person to be compliant, instead of remaining unyielding and obstinate.

We learn that when Bnei Yisrael committed the Sin of the Golden Calf, Hashem told Moshe

< 232 >

(Shemos 32), "Go, descend, for your people ...
have become corrupt ... I have seen this people
and ... it is a stiff-necked people ... and I shall
annihilate them."

HaGaon HaRav Shalom Mordechai Schwadron
points out that Hashem focused on the nation's
obstinacy and stubbornness, and not the sin
itself. Rashi notes that they turned their backs on
those who reproached them and refused to listen
to them. The act of confession is diametrically
opposed to that response and indicates sincere
contrition for one's misdeeds.

It takes great courage to tread this path, but
therein lies one's salvation.

< 233 >

Step Six

Were entirely ready to have G-d remove all these defects of character.

Our nation is mandated to look forward, ever hopeful and positive, rather than lamenting over past mistakes and failures, or becoming weighed down by previous disappointments or setbacks.

The Torah tells us *(Bereishis 19:26)* that when Lot and his family were saved from the destruction of Sodom and Amora, Lot's wife looked back, behind her, and became a pillar of salt. The commentaries ask: Why did Lot's wife deserve such a severe punishment for looking over her shoulder? It is explained that Hashem was providing an opportunity for a fresh beginning in life, the wherewithal to turn over a new leaf, and Lot's wife chose to have another look at her past, to reconsider what she was leaving behind. She was reluctant to look forward to the future.

An individual's unwillingness to separate from the past can certainly impede his future success. The Torah true philosophy discourages focusing on one's earlier errors, his debacles and fiascos. No matter how many unsuccessful attempts a person has made to accomplish something, he should continue to persevere in his efforts. He should always look forward with hope and anticipation that he will triumph and be successful.

The Mishnah in *Yuma (8:9)* states: Who is it before whom you are purified? And who is it

< 234 >

that purifies you? Your Father who is in Heaven, as it says *(Yechezkel 36:25)*, "I will sprinkle clean water upon you and you shall be clean" and it further says *(Yirmiyah 17:13)*, "Oh Hashem, Hope of Israel!"

Our sages tell us that there are two forms of purification from sin. The impure person enters the *mikvah* and immerses himself in its holy waters; or the impure person remains in his place and pure water flows over him. These two modes actually define two different types of individuals who seek to do *teshuvah*. One person is forceful and decisive; he is able to work on himself and draw closer to Hashem. He goes to the *mikvah* and initiates the purification process. The other person is weak and hesitant; he is distant from Hashem and needs His help to strengthen their bond. He is passive, so the clean water is sprinkled on him by others. Inert, he finds it difficult to eradicate his flawed qualities on his own; he needs Hashem's intervention to assist his efforts to purify his soul.

Indeed, the Talmud confirms *(Yuma 38b)*, "If he comes to purify himself he is helped."

< 235 >

Step Seven

Humbly asked Him to remove our shortcomings.

It is well known that every human being has shortcomings; no one is perfect. Nevertheless, these frailties do not preclude one's responsibility to behave in accordance with the Torah. Flawed personality traits only present a greater challenge to do the right thing.

Personal growth is a lifetime effort. The Vilna Gaon notes *(Even Shleimah)* that man's main purpose in life is to relentlessly strive to eradicate his bad habits. Moreover, Hashem constantly presents us with opportunities and challenges to help us achieve our potential. One must always evoke the Talmudic dictum *(Sanhedrin 37a)*, "*Bishvili nivra ha'olam* – the world was created for me." Rashi explains that each person is considered as important as the entire world.

Hashem used the Torah as a blueprint for the creation of the world and that is the purpose of the world's creation. Torah upholds the world.

The Rambam writes in *Hilchos Teshuvah (7:3)* that character refinement is an important part of the *teshuvah* process. It is a prerequisite for the mastery of Torah. Ideally, we should repair our character flaws through Torah study by internalizing its moral teachings. Torah study teaches one how to live.

We acknowledge that we have character deficits and negative personality traits such as jealousy, rage, anger, selfishness, stinginess, and greed,

< 236 >

and we ask Hashem to help us eliminate or redirect those instincts and impulses. For example, if a person sought honor for himself, he requests Hashem to redirect his urge so that he desires to pursue the honor of Hashem. If he indulged in acts that are prohibited by the Torah, he prays to Hashem to be empowered so that he achieves more control of his inclinations and drives.

We are instructed (Rambam, *Hilchos Temurah* *4:13)* that the *mitzvos,* in fact, help us to correct our negative character traits and achieve refinement and perfection of one's character.

< 237 >

Step Eight

Made a list of all persons we had harmed, and became willing to make amends to them all.

These are people – perhaps in one's own family – who have been negatively affected by the addict's behavior. He surely set a wrong example for others, and may have even influenced someone to join him in his addiction. People were hurt, embarrassed, or suffered mental anguish because of his/her addiction. Money or property may have been stolen.

The Rambam states in *Hilchos Teshuvah (2:9)* that sins between man and his fellow man are not forgiven by Hashem. The absolution must come from the one who has been aggrieved. The individual who sinned must make restitution for that which he is liable. He must also ask forgiveness from the individual(s) he has harmed. He must ask to be forgiven for any type of act that he may have committed against another, whether it was a physical, verbal or financial act.

Putting in writing the names of those who have been negatively affected by his injurious activities is a reflective undertaking that can effectively evoke and intensify true feelings of remorse on the part of the addict.

The Talmud tells us that Shaul HaMelech who sinned with one transgression – he did not destroy all of Amalek – lost his kingdom. David HaMelech, on the other hand, who transgressed twice, was pardoned and remained king.

< 238 >

It would seem that Shaul was treated much more harshly than David, especially in light of the greater severity of David's sins, postulates the Maharsha. He explains, however, that it was the contrast of their responses that determined their ultimate fate. When Nassan HaNavi rebuked David HaMelech, following the sin of Batsheva, David responded, "I have sinned to Hashem." Although Shaul too replied to Shmuel HaNavi, "I have sinned, violating the word of Hashem," he continued to justify why he had acted the way he did. Shaul tried to transfer his culpability, rather than take full responsibility as David did. In that sense, Shaul HaMelech's *teshuvah* was not complete.

Taking responsibility for one's actions is a significant step in the *teshuvah* process and a therapeutic course of action. In addition, asking for forgiveness is intrinsically a humbling act and therefore serves as an atonement by and of itself.

< 239 >

Step Nine

Made direct amends to such people wherever possible, except when to do so would injure them or others.

Shalom, peace, is an important concept in Judaism. It is emphasized constantly in our *tefillos* (prayer) and we conclude every *Shemone Esrei* with the prayer, "He Who makes peace in His heights, may He make peace upon us, and upon all Israel."

The Medrash *(Vayikra Rabbah)* comments on the *pasuk* in *Tehillim (34:15)*, "Love peace and pursue it," and notes that unlike other *mitzvos*, peace is different. It is not a passive *mitzvah*, which one waits to perform if the opportunity presents itself. Rather, one is obligated to leave no stone unturned in his pursuit of peace. One has to actively remove the obstacles that prevent the promotion of peace, go out of his way to encourage and support peace – whether in his own relationship with others, or anyone else's associations.

The Torah tells us *(Bamidbar 20:29)* that when Aharon died "the entire House of Israel wept for thirty days." Rashi explains that the grief was universal because if there was a quarrel between two individuals or between husband and wife Aharon would make peace between them.

Furthermore, states the Rambam *(Hilchos Chanukah, Chapter 4)*, "Great is peace, for the entire Torah was given to make peace in the world."

< 240 >

Nevertheless, one must be careful to avoid transgressing the Torah prohibition of, "You shall not cause pain to your fellow man" *(Vayikra 25:17)*, known as *ona'as devarim*. For example, if one harmed someone else in any way, but his "victim" is unaware of it, it may be counterproductive to inform him of that act. It is not for naught that we sometimes say, "Ignorance is bliss," for it is not always prudent for the addict to unburden himself and alleviate his own pain, at the expense of his oblivious victim.

The Chofetz Chaim gives us sage advice that we should not assess what is hurtful to another by our own standards but rather by evaluating the other person's sensitivities.

< 241 >

Step Ten

Continued to take personal inventory and when we were wrong promptly admitted it.

A personal inventory includes more than taking stock of one's present situation. It means reviewing the past and making certain that amends have been made for misdeeds committed in the past.

Rabbeinu Yonah, in his classic *Shaarei Teshuvah*, comments on the importance of immediately admitting one's mistakes and making the appropriate reparations. He presents the instance of a group of prisoners who are languishing in jail. One day, the warden forgets to lock the prison cells and all the prisoners flee, except for one inmate who is too lazy to get up. When the warden returns, he rebukes the detainee, "You fool! Why didn't you escape when you had the opportunity?"

This is an illustration of a person who procrastinates and doesn't hasten to repent, explains Rabbeinu Yonah.

A personal inventory also requires going even further back in one's personal history and analyzing the digressions, missteps and wrong turns that brought one to this point in life.

Our sages tell us that every person has a specific mission in life. Every

< 242 >

individual is born with unique talents, traits, strengths, and weaknesses specifically designed to help him fulfill his special mission.

By re-evaluating his life, a person is given the opportunity to take note of his mistakes and makes the necessary adjustments. He is able to identify his bad moves and "recalculate" the route that will reconnect him to Hashem and to his ultimate realization of his *tafkid*, his life mission.

< 243 >

Step Eleven

Sought through prayer and meditation to improve our conscious contact with G-d *as we understood Him*, praying only for knowledge of His will for us and the power to carry that out.

Prayer is the service of the heart. It is the medium through which we praise Hashem and thank Him for His blessings. But it is also the vehicle of our requests and pleas for understanding, success and good health.

The Shalah HaKadosh explains that there are many initiatives one can incorporate in his life to promote sincere prayer and improve one's bond with Hashem:

- Learning Torah diligently and acclimating oneself to praising Hashem

- Designating a quiet place which offers privacy and allows one to focus his thoughts in prayer

- Appreciating the unique opportunity to "speak with Hashem" and fervently appealing to Hashem to grant his physical and spiritual needs

- Contemplating one's personal insignificance relative to the greatness of his Creator and recognizing all the good that Hashem has done for him, prior to beginning his prayers

< 244 >

Shir HaShirim Rabbah states there is no better means of approaching Hashem than in prayer.

The Zohar notes (*Tikunim 18*) that when a person utters words of *tefillah*, the birds spread their wings and receive them, as it says (*Koheles 10:20*), "For the bird of the skies may carry the sound." Hashem then takes these words and uses them to build new worlds, as it says (*Yeshayah 66:22*), "For just as the new heavens and the new earth that I will make will endure before Me – the word of Hashem – so will your offspring and your name endure." Thus we establish a unique partnership with Hashem.

Rabbi Nachman of Breslov says, "Prayers truly from the heart open all the doors in heaven."

< 245 >

Step Twelve

Having had a spiritual awakening as the result of these steps, we tried to carry this message to others, and to practice these principles in all our affairs.

The Talmud *(Shavuos 39a)* teaches that all Jews are responsible for one another. The concept of *areivus* (responsibility) is a fundamental Torah principle, for the Torah was given to the Jewish nation at Har Sinai, to the people as a whole. Perforce, it is the obligation of each and every Jew to ensure his own fulfillment of the *mitzvos* as well as to promote the performance of the *mitzvos* by all the members of the Jewish people.

We learn that the Torah command of loving Hashem includes the obligation of *kiruv,* bringing our fellow Jews closer to Hashem (Rambam, *Sefer HaMitzvos, Mitzvas Aseh 3).* The Rambam notes that people who never learned about Torah and *mitzvos* are considered like children who were kidnapped and raised among non-Jews *(tinokos shenishbu).* Such individuals must be encouraged with words of love to return to the path of Torah.

As we seek to guide someone in their return to the ways of Torah, it is important to bear in mind our sages' principle *(Sotah 47a),* "Let the left hand thrust away and the right hand draw [him] close." HaGaon HaRav Simcha Wasserman notes that if we simply push away the sinner with both hands, it only creates a greater distance between him and Hashem and sends him further along his ill-chosen path. But if we simultaneously draw the sinner close, we are effectively turning

< 246 >

him 180 degrees and steering him away from the dangerous road he has been traveling.

Whoever helps a person to return to the path of Torah achieves a level of spirituality that is three points higher than the level of others, says the Zohar. Such an individual subjugates the *sitra achra* (the forces of evil); he elevates the honor of Hashem; and he affirmatively affects the existence of the world. He will also merit to see his children's children; he will merit *olam hazeh* and *olam haba* (this world and the next); and others will not have the power to judge him, neither in this world nor in the next. He will enter the twelve Heavenly Gates with no detractors.

Our sages tell us *(Shabbos 31a)* that when man will be led to judgment before the Heavenly Court, among the questions he will be asked is whether he established times for learning. HaGaon HaRav Mordechai Gifter explains that "times for learning" is not quantifiable. Rather, he says, it represents an all inclusive life of Torah that permeates every aspect of daily living. A person will be questioned whether Torah was an integral component of his conduct at work and at home. Judgment will be passed on whether Torah served as a guideline in all his recreational practices and professional dealings.

< 247 >

Epilogue

Man has been veritably placed in the midst of a raging battle. For all of the affairs of the world, whether for the good or for the bad, are trials to a man: Poverty on the one hand and wealth on the other, serenity on the one hand and suffering on the other, so that the battle rages from both sides. If he is victorious on all sides, he will be the "Whole Man."

(R' Moshe Chaim Luzzatto, Mesilas Yesharim)

The "raging battle" of life surrounds us each moment of each day. Good and bad, suffering and serenity, health and illness, all challenge us alike. So how should a person react to life's tests – to *nisyonos*? Why, indeed, are we subjected to these never-ending tests? And perhaps most important, how can we emerge victorious in this lifelong battle, so that we become, as the *Mesilas Yesharim* (Path of the Just) says, "whole"?

The Force Behind the Challenge – and Our Power to Overcome It

There is a force within us that creates these challenges. It brings the rich to miserliness and the poor to despair, the suffering to doubt and the untroubled to complacency. It possesses the power to take each human condition and turn it into a test of faith and strength. It is the *yetzer hara* (the Evil Inclination), the unwelcome guest in the soul of every human being.

There will come a time when the *yetzer hara* will lose its power. The Talmud tells us that at the end of days, Hashem will slaughter the *yetzer hara* in front of the *tzaddikim* (the righteous)

< 248 >

and in front of the *resha'im* (the wicked). In the *olam ha'emes* (the World of Truth) the *yetzer hara* will appear in its true form, unmasked by human misinterpretation. Still, it will appear in different forms to different people.

The *yetzer hara* will appear to the *tzaddik* as a mighty mountain, and to the *rasha* as a thin hair-like strand. But in the World of Truth, both the righteous and the wicked will know beyond doubt that what he sees is the very force that has challenged him all life through. And interestingly, the Talmud tells us that both will cry at the sight.

How can it be, asks Rabbi Kolonymus Kalman, the Me'or V'Shemesh, that the same entity – the *yetzer hara* – will appear so differently to different people? How can the *tzaddik* see it as a mountain and the *rasha* as a hair?

It is because each person will see the *yetzer hara* as the challenges with which he was presented. The *tzaddik*, who throughout his life faced difficult tests, will see the mountain of challenges he overcame. He will recall the trials and tests he faced, each one meted out to him according to his ability to overcome it. He will understand the power of his faith, and the way each test strengthened it to massive proportions. And when faced with the magnitude of his battle and the massive efforts he exerted – the *har govoha*, the mighty mountain – he will cry, overwhelmed with emotion at his success.

The *rasha*, too, will see the *yetzer hara* as the challenges he has encountered. But his challenges were smaller. Chazal tell us, *"Ein Hakadosh Baruch Hu bo b'trunyo* – Hashem does not challenge a person with something he cannot handle." The wicked person was never challenged beyond his ability. Although he may have faced tests that seemed mighty at the time, in the *olam ha'emes* he will be forced to recognize that his trials were not difficult at all. They were merely a thin strand of challenge.

< 249 >

He may remember the time his elderly mother asked him to help her cross the street.

"I can't do it," he might have thought at the time. "How can I be seen crossing her? It's so embarrassing." Or, perhaps he thought that the time was inconvenient. Or that his mother was taking advantage of him. Whatever his excuse, it seemed perfectly valid at the time. But in the World of Truth, excuses will fade, and he will be forced to face the painful truth – that he could have conquered his *yetzer hara*.

He will understand for the first time that all of his trials could have been so easily overcome – it would have been as simple as stepping over his miniscule *yetzer hara*. He will weep in remorse, but it will be too late. All he will be able to do then is cry for the battle lost forever.

Such is life. No matter how difficult the situation, how insurmountable the odds, we do have the power to overcome life's challenges. The *nisyonos* that are sent our way are for our benefit. They spur us on to greater faith, and to greater depth of character and soul.

Nisyonos – the Impetus for Personal Growth

We ask Hashem each morning that we not be brought to *nisayon* – that we not be enticed to sin. But we were put in this world primarily to overcome *nisyonos*. *Nisyonos* allow us to grow, to become better. Why, then, do we ask to be spared from challenge?

The Michtav M'Eliyahu answers that we ask only that we not be tested severely. We ask that we be presented only with *nisyonos* that are not difficult to overcome, because prevailing over *nisyonos* can be difficult. In fact, the word *nisayon* stems from the word *nes* – miracle. The fact that we can and do

< 250 >

overcome these challenges is miraculous. But Hashem provides the strength, and we invest the effort, reaping the rewards of success forever.

Still, we need to be constantly on guard for new *nisyonos*, and recognize them as such, for they confront us at every turn in life. They arise in business. They arise at home. And often, one does not even realize that he has been tested.

There are the big tests – the man who must choose between *mincha* and a multi-million dollar business deal, the patient who tries to find faith at the door to the operating room, the widow who must come to grips with her loss.

And there are the daily tests – the mother who needs to control her anger in the face of chaos, the desire to slide into a parking spot before someone else, the less-than-kosher garment or forms of entertainment.

We pray that we be spared the big tests of life. And we ask that we be granted the strength to overcome even the smaller ones. Because they, too, are part of the Divine Plan, and it is the smaller, less-obvious challenges, that prepare us for the mountainous ones.

A People Equipped for the Challenge

Klal Yisrael is called a stiff-necked people – *am keshei oref* (*Shemos 34:9*). The *tzaddik* Rebbe Arye Levine asks: How could Moshe Rabbeinu, who defended the Jewish people through so many trials, call Bnei Yisrael a stiff-necked people? How can he refer to Klal Yisrael in such a derogatory manner?

R' Levine answers that the name is not derogatory. Rather, Moshe Rabbeinu meant to say that we are stiff-necked in our service of Hashem. We are stubborn, but we

< 251 >

direct our stubbornness to the fight for spirituality. We are fiercely determined to win Hashem's battles, whether or not we understand them. We are an *am keshei oref* – a stiff-necked people. And that is one secret of our success.

Faith and Challenge

There are times when the challenges we face are clear as day. During those times, we can comprehend our challenges, and confidently overcome them, guided by our steadfast faith. Those are the times during the day. Those are the times we refer to in the *Krias Shema* of *shacharis*, the morning prayer, when, after declaring our faith we say *emes v'yatziv* – true and firm. We can positively confirm that what we have said is true, for we have seen it.

But then there is the night – the times when our *emunah* must come from deep within, for we do not have our faith strengthened by the obvious. Those are the times we refer to each night, after *Krias Shema*, when we say *emes ve'emunah* – true and faithful, for at times when Hashem's Hand is hidden from us, we still remain faithful – though we must remain in the dark, and cannot understand His ways.

When a Jew retains his *emunah* in the darkest times, he affirms his faith during the day as well. He can say the words of *Tehillim*, "*Nasata l'rei'echo nes l'hisnosess* – You have given a banner to those who fear You, that it may be displayed." The word *nes* can mean a test, for when a person passes a *nisayon*, he proudly carries the banner of Hashem.

Sometimes a person becomes ensnared in his *aveiros* and he feels trapped. His soul longs to be close to Hashem and to experience His love on a deeper level, but he has drifted far from the Torah's path. When the individual finally succeeds in extricating himself from his dire predicament, he emerges with a deeper appreciation for the King of the world. His love is

< 252 >

more intense than that of the *tzaddik*, the righteous person, who has never gone astray and has never been enslaved in captivity.

The Baal Shem Tov explains this with a parable of a king who had two sons. Once when they went into battle, one of the sons was taken prisoner. It was many months before the king's son managed to escape his captors and return home to the palace. Obviously his joy and appreciation to be home, in the loving embrace of his father, the king, is much more intense than that of the other son who had always remained at his father's side. Being incarcerated had intensified his gratitude and affection for his father, the king.

Teshuvah is the key that releases one from the bondage of his *aveiros.* Man is tested every day with various *nisyonos,* and there are many people who fail. Regardless of the depths to which the person has fallen, and no matter the subjugation to which he is subjected, one should never despair. The wise person will understand that he is being tested by Hashem. He will fortify his spirit, reach higher and free himself.

< 253 >

Postscript

Very often, successful treatment of an addiction must include the intervention of a mental health professional, whether psychiatrist and/or psychologist or social worker. Of course, when seeking help, one should preferably find a qualified professional who specializes in addiction counseling. It is also of paramount importance to work with an individual whose ideologies and beliefs are in sync with the Jewish patient's values and thinking.

HaGaon Rav Moshe Feinstein notes in his responsa *(Igros Moshe 57)* that although one may be referred to a medical doctor who is an atheist or heretic, there is usually minimal, if any, exchange of philosophical thoughts in such intervention. In an exclusive medical situation, the illness is basically healed by a course of medicinal therapy or medical protocols. If, however, the doctor resorted to incantations or the like (chanting or uttering words purporting to have magical power) it would be forbidden to use his services.

On the other hand, writes Rav Feinstein, consulting psychologists or psychiatrists whose main course of therapy is the communication and exchange of thoughts and ideas, which may include all types of heresy and impropriety in language or thought, is an entirely different matter. Since it is necessary for the patient to discuss the different dilemmas he faces because of his challenges, there is a serious concern that the counseling may not be appropriate for the Jewish patient.

In conclusion, Rav Feinstein concedes that it may be possible to rely on a doctor who is an expert in his field and promises the patient not to say anything contrary to his faith, or not in consonance with the Torah perspective, since he is honor-bound by the Hippocratic Oath. Nevertheless, optimally, one should seek a therapist who is empathetic

< 254 >

to Jewish values and whose morals and ethics are in agreement with a Torah way of life.

For consultations, please email
contacttherav@gmail.com.

< 255 >

About the Author

Rabbi Dovid Goldwasser is known for his exceptional ability to captivate and inspire audiences worldwide. He disseminates Torah to thousands through the daily Morning Chizuk program on New Jersey's WFMU and his weekly discourse on the Torah portion on New York's WSNR. A highly sought-after and renowned speaker, the Rav of Brooklyn's Congregation Bnei Yitzchok has traveled extensively throughout the United States, Israel and Europe, galvanizing audiences from every background with his eloquence and dynamism.

Rabbi Goldwasser provides reassurance and inspiration, counseling young people, couples and families globally. For more than twenty years, he has been a leading proponent in the community for the prompt recognition of addictions and eating disorders, and their proper treatment. He works closely with medical personnel and mental health professionals, facilities, and their patients, and has written extensively on addictions and eating disorders.

Rabbi Goldwasser has authored over a dozen books, focusing on different themes, ranging from insights into the weekly Torah portion, to first-hand stories of faith and encouragement, and the Torah perspective on mental health issues. Rabbi Goldwasser also writes on a broad range of key issues of relevance for today's society as a weekly columnist in the Jewish Press; is a contributing writer for many publications; serves as a faculty member of Touro Lander College; and is an acknowledged expert in educational concerns.

< 256 >